Aging without aging

James Defares

Aging without aging

*THE PRACTICAL SCIENCE
OF 'REACHING 120
AND STAYING 60'*

Uitgeverij Aspekt

AGING WITHOUT AGING
© James Defares
© 2015 Uitgeverij ASPEKT
Amersfoortsestraat 27, 3769 AD Soesterberg, Nederland
info@uitgeverijaspekt.nl-http://www.uitgeverijaspekt.nl

Omslagontwerp: Thomas Wunderink
Binnenwerk: Thomas Wunderink

ISBN: 9789461537331
NUR: 860

Alle rechten voorbehouden. Niets van deze uitgave mag worden verveelvoudigd, opgeslagen in een geautomatiseerd gegevensbestand of openbaar gemaakt, in enige vorm of op enige wijze, hetzij elektronisch, mechanisch, door fotokopieën, opnamen of enig andere manier, zonder voorafgaande toestemming van de uitgever.

Voorzover het maken van kopieën uit deze uitgave is toegestaan op grond van artikel 16B Auteurswet 1912 j° het Besluit van 20 juni 1974, St.b. 351, zoals gewijzigd bij het Besluit van 23 augustus 1985, St.b. 471 en artikel 17 Auteurswet 1912, dient men de daarvoor wettelijk verschuldigde vergoedingen te voldoen aan de Stichting Reprorecht (postbus 882, 1180 AW, Amstelveen). Voor het overnemen van gedeelte(n) van deze uitgave in bloemlezingen, readers, en andere compilatiewerken (artikel 16 Auteurswet 1912), dient men zich tot de uitgever te wenden.

Contents

Preface		7
1	Is man a meat-eater?	11
2	The anti-aging diet	15
3	How much protein a day?	23
4	Sugar: the White Death	27
5	Metformin: the 'youth pill' + Medical appendix	34
6	Overweight and cancer + Medical appendix	43
7	Metformin and cancer prevention	52
8	Your body weight and cancer risk	55
9	Carbohydrates, insulin and Alzheimer's disease + Medical appendix	56
10	About baking, broiling, cheese and breakfast cereals: careful! + Medical appendix	61
11	Cholesterol, saturated fats, statins and your heart	67
12	Resveratrol: life-extender and CR-mimetic? + Medical appendix	80
13	Telomeres: the 'time clock' of your life	86
14	TA-65: the only real "rejuvenation pill"	93
15	L-Arginine: protection against atherosclerosis and heart attacks	97
16	Atherosclerosis: chronic subclinical 'scurvy' + Medical appendix	103
17	Atherosclerosis: the 'silent killer'	116
18	Exercise and its benefits	122
19	Estrogen replacement after the menopause?	123
19A	May women who have had breast cancer take estrogen (ERT)?	137
20	Testosteron, the hormone of life	152
21	The birth control pill is very harmful	160
22	The fundamental cause of aging: the telomere	164
23	Secondary causes of aging	170
24	The most important anti-aging antioxidants	184
25	Diabetes and insulin therapy	190
26	Are we our brain?	193
27	Meditation and aging	197
28	Smoking, a deadly sin	200
29	Losing weight: fast and permanent	202
30	Stress and aging	205
31	Bald? A matter of choice	208
32	How to protect myself against cancer	210
33	DHEA memory and Alzheimer's disease + Medical appendix	214
34	Growth hormone: obsolete	228
35	Chelation therapy for narrowed arteries	230

36	Osteoarthritis (prevention) and glucosamine	241
37	The libido pill	244
38	Supplements against telomere shrinkage	251
39	Nocturnal leg cramps	255
40	Irregular heartbeats and pig's heart valve: matters of the heart	257
41	The sleeping pill and eternal sleep	262
42	C60 doubles the lifespan of rats	265
43	Bad marriage, bad health	270

Preface

This book has been written for anyone above eighteen. It is a practical guide for a healthier and longer life. Although the information presented is scientifically based this is definitely not a 'scientific' book intended for readers with an academic background.

Anyone, from the babysitter to the lawyer, will be able to read and understand the contents without any difficulty. Technical information intended for the 'expert' has been put in frames. This should in no way distract the reader and may even bolster his faith in the reliability of the material.

The purpose of this book is to offer the reader a practical guide for staying healthy today and tomorrow, to slow down aging and extend lifespan. That this is a realistic goal already follows from such statistics as those of the CBS (Dutch *Central Bureau of Statistics*) which show that college graduates live seven years longer than blue-collar workers and while the 'healthy years' extend to the age of 72 in college graduates they do not exceed 53 years in blue-collar workers: a difference of 19 years.

This illustrates that the duration (quantity) of 'healthy years' (quality) is not just determined by our genes, but can be drastically influenced by circumstances, lifestyle and other factors.

In order to express the central idea behind this book I would venture to say that if one starts to 'act' at middle age or earlier according to the principles and 'tools' presented in this book life-expectancy in relation to that of blue-collar workers could be extended to 20 years and the 'healthy years' to 40 years.

More concretely: many a reader who has been living foolishly thus far will be able to live at least 20 years longer and enjoy an additional 40 years of 'healthy years' if he/she takes the advice given in this book to heart.

As the contents of this book are based on scientific findings, a proper subtitle would be "The practical science of bio-aging and bio-rejuvenation."

What is the cause of aging and death?
The aging of the body cell. We are as young and as old as our 50 trillion body cells. These cells have a genetically determined (but adjustable) time clock: the telomere (see chapter 13), a piece of DNA. The fundamental strategy is to reset the hand of this time clock and/or to slow down the speed of this ticking time clock (chapters 10 and 11). All this sounds mysterious but everything will be revealed in this book.

On the basis of animal trials with different species, ranging from rats to dogs, in which they are put on a 'hunger diet' (30 per cent less calories than they would normally consume) and live 20 to 30 per cent longer in excellent health (less cancer, less diabetes, etc.) we now know that a very important factor for a longer and healthier life is keeping the insulin- and glucose blood level(s) low.

The aging process is accelerated by the degree of atherosclerosis, the cause of death of more than 60 per cent of the population in the West (stroke, heart attack, etc.). Hence a great deal of attention is given to this condition which affects us all. Beyond fifty a sex hormone deficiency (oestrogen in the female, testosterone in the male), often occurs, as a result of which the aging process goes in overdrive. Correcting these deficits by the use of bio-identical hormones greatly retards the process of aging and its manifestations (osteoporosis, loss of height, etc.).

Measures for cancer prevention (1 in 3 people get cancer) also come up for discussion.

Protection against so-called oxygen free radicals, very harmful by-products of cell respiration, constitutes an important component of the anti-aging strategy.

Apart from the recommended supplements and other preparations, lifestyle and eating habits play a crucial role in influencing the aging process by the abovementioned mechanisms.

A single example: overweight leads to high insulin- and glucose levels and so accelerates aging and increases mortality risk. Chronic stress ages the cells by speeding up the ticking time clock (shortening of telomeres, chapter 13). Too much sugar and carbohydrates speed up aging and increase the risk of heart attacks. These are just some examples of the interaction between lifestyle and the fundamental processes underlying bio-aging, that are fully discussed in this handbook for 'living longer while staying young.'

Chapter 1

Is man a meat-eater?

When you own a car you should know whether it runs on gasoline, diesel or LPG. It is the same with your body. Is man by nature a vegetarian, meat-eater, or omnivore? For the rational choice of our optimal diet the answer to this question is of paramount importance.

The opposite of a meat-eater is not necessarily a vegetarian. It could be a fish-eater and even an ostrich-eater. Here the term meat refers to meat from quadrupeds, in particular cows, pigs and sheep.

Let me start with a few preliminary remarks. In books on vegetarianism it is often argued that, on the basis of the shape and structure of fossil teeth and molars, that our ancestors of some 100,000 years ago were herbivores. So, we – according to these books - are herbivores by nature. It is a weak and in fact superfluous argument. We do not look at fossils from prehistoric times to prove that the lion is a meat-eater by nature. Even if no one had ever seen a lion (in action) one would on the basis of a single molar of a contemporary lion conclude that it is a carnivore. We do not have to, no we should not in fact, go back in time. We should just look at some characteristics of animals (including man) that are alive today. Is our organism constructed for meat consumption or for a vegetable diet? This is a meaningful question. After all, before you put fuel into the tank of your car you should know whether the car has been constructed to run on gasoline, diesel or LPG.

Schematically we may - with intermediate forms - divide mammals on the basis of their eating habits into three categories: carnivores (meat-eaters), herbivores (plant-eaters), and frugivores (fruit-eaters).

Among the primates, to which man belongs, we find meat-eaters, plant-eaters and fruit-eaters. The smaller the species - for example the lemur - the higher the percentage of carnivores. The greatest primate – the orang-utan (literally wood man) from Borneo and Sumatra is a fruit-eater or frugivore. The durian, a fruit bigger than a football, which, in Indonesia is also a delicacy for man, is the main source of protein for the orang-utan. Only after copying the art from his father for years, the young ape learns to find the fruit in the huge trees that even orang-utans find hard to climb and to break open the tough cactus-like skin of the fruit.

Most big primates are mainly fruit-eaters that get their protein from leaves, small animals and insects. But what about the chimpanzee, our nearest cousin? According to DNA-research only 3 per cent of the DNA of both species is non-identical, while the DNA[1] differences between chimp and man are less than between chimp and gorilla. Does it follow from this that man is, like the chimpanzee, a fruit-eater by nature? No, it is suggestive, but not conclusive.[2]

If we draw an equilateral triangle with the pure meat-eater at the left base angle, the pure plant-eater at the right base angle and the fruit-eater at the top angle then most species of the order of primates are located on the right side or within the triangle close to the right side. This indicates that the majority of the gibbons and the great apes are a mixture of frugivores (fruit and seed eaters) and foliovores, also termed herbivores (leaf, flower and bark eaters). Is that proof of the true nature of man? No, because man is, of course, - also with regard to adaptability – unique.

For a definitive answer to this question biologists focus on everything related to digestion, like the anatomy of the teeth, the stomach, the intestines, the digestive enzymes, etc. If we look at the intestines of mammals, we notice that in the carnivore the small intestine – where the absorption of nutrients takes place - strongly dominates, while the large intestine (colon) is either quite short or entirely absent.

---

1   DNA is the acronym for des-oxy-ribo-nucleic acid, the blue print of life in which the genetic information is stored. This very long molecule (2 meters long when unravelled) is de basis of our genes and chromosomes.
2   Baboons and macaques consume 70 to 80 per cent of their food as fruit. But besides leaves and roots they also eat animals, including small mammals. The same holds for chimpanzees.

Pure folivores (herbivores), like horses, cows, etc., need a big compartment for the bacterial fermentation of the cellulose membrane of leaves and grasses. This is achieved by a long colon and caecum and to a lesser extent by leaves-eating primates like the gorilla, the howling monkey, etc.

Between those two extremes lie - anatomically speaking - the fruit-eating primates. The stomach and especially the colon are in frugivores considerably larger than in the carnivores or frugivores, because of the necessity to digest fruit and young leaves. The digestive tract of man lies closer to that of foliovores and frugivores than to that of carnivores (meat-eaters). But we aren't there yet. Because of large differences in body size a correction must be applied, which is referred to by the mathematical expression *dimensional analysis*.

The result is a graphic representation – the multidimensional scheme – in which the place of man is clearly shown. Don't get alarmed. It looks complicated, but all you have to do is cast a glance at the figure below.

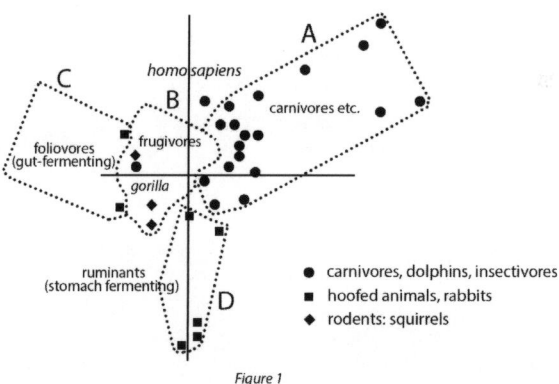

Figure 1

It looks like a map with four areas, A, B, C and D. In A are mainly the carnivores (faunivores), in B the frugivores (including many primates), C contains the gut-fermenting foliovores, like horses and apes and in D we find the stomach fermenting foliovores like ruminants and Columbine monkeys.

Where is man located?
The position of man in figure 1 falls outside the four areas mentioned, to wit, above the boundary between the carnivores and the frugivores (fruiteaters). This important study is based on 80 different mammal species (including many primates). The study shows that man by nature (because of his build) is not a meat-eater, nor a fruit-eater, but is between these two, or better, towers above them.

It is incorrect to say that man is a vegetarian by nature, just as it is incorrect to state that he is a carnivore. So, is man an omnivore? An omnivore is an animal that eats (large) quantities of meat as well as (large) quantities of leaves, etc. This combination is for physiological reasons impossible. So, the concept 'omnivore' does not exist as a technical *term* in biology. Thanks to the discovery of the use of fire and the techniques of food processing one could regard man as the only omnivore. The position of *homo sapiens in* the graph reflects the unique adaptability of man.

Chapter 2

The anti-aging diet

In chapters 4-8 I have discussed at length that high glucose– and insulin levels are harmful for your health and promote the aging process as well as the development of geriatric illnesses (cancer, Alzheimer, diabetes, etc.).

So a diet low in sugar and carbohydrates is thus far healthier than a carbohydrates-rich diet with a lot of bread, rice, potatoes or pasta.

Does a diet low in carbs necessarily mean a protein-rich diet like the Atkins diet?

No, since a 'protein-rich' diet is also unhealthy, one reason being that most of the protein is then derived from meat or dairy products.

But what should one then eat for heaven's sake? Carb-rich is not allowed, protein–rich is not allowed either, a diet rich in fats is awful and unhealthy?

The answer is simple and primitive: the Paleo diet. The Paleo diet or cave man diet, Stone-age diet (Paleo = prehistoric). So, indeed, the Paleo diet means to eat like our ancestors in the Stone-age, between one million years ago and 10,000 years ago, the start of the agrarian era.

But while the proponents of the Paleo diet base their arguments on our one million years old genetic adaptation to the available food for the primitive hunter-gatherer, the diet that I recommend is purely based on its merits for a longer and healthier life.

In order to give the child a name and a certain degree of respectability I will refer to it as **the Paleo diet, simply because of the close relationship between the two.**

Coincidence or biological 'logic', but the healthiest diet turns out to correspond closely with the diet of the hunter-gatherer, the caveman.

Let me start with a brief outline of the historic background of the Paleo diet, developed, not by "New-Age sectarians" but by serious medical scientists.

Paleo diet

At first sight the Paleo diet looks pretty awful to some: it mainly consists of vegetables, fruit, meat, fish, mushrooms, roots and nuts. It excludes grains, dairy products, potatoes, rice, bread, pasta, etc.

The emphasis is on vegetables, fruits, root crops and nuts. The amount of meat or fish allowed varies with the views of the different researchers in the field of the so-called evolutionary medicine. This is the branch of medicine based on the evolutionary development of man and his DNA.

The Paleo diet, popularized in the second half of the seventies by the gastroenterologist Dr. Walter Voeglin, is supported by archaeological evidence from the Palaeolithic and Neolithic (recent 10,000 years) periods.[3]

A powerful argument in favour of the Paleo diet is that present-day (primitive) populations that eat according to the traditions of their distant forebears, like on some islands in New Guinea (e.g. Kitava) do not suffer from 'diseases of civilization' like heart disease, diabetes, hypertension, atherosclerosis, etc.

Statistical studies in which test persons follow either the Paleo diet or a different 'healthy' diet (Mediterranean diet, anti-diabetes type 2 diet, etc.) have confirmed the superiority of the Paleo diet. An example is presented in the frame

> A clinical randomized, cross-over study compared the Paleo diet with frequently prescribed diet for diabetes type-2. The Paleo diet resulted in lower values of HBA1c, triacylglycerol, diastolic pressure, body mass index (BMI) and higher HDL cholesterol than the anti-diabetes diet.

---

3   Richards, M.P., "A brief review of the archaeological evidence for Palaeolithic and Neolithic subsistence." European Journal of Clinical Nutrition, 56, 1270, 2002.

In the various variants of the Paleo diet we find large differences in the plant-animal ratio, or the percentage of meat as a source of protein. For us this is inconsequential as we leave the Paleo diet and restrict ourselves to the 'ideal' anti-aging diet that happens to correspond with a certain variant of the Paleo diet. Just to 'baptize the child', to give it a name with a respectable history, we shall call it the Paleo diet, or why not a step further, the Paleo anti-aging diet.

The Paleo anti-aging diet
Man is what he eats. In German it sounds better: **Der Mensch ist was er ißt.** Biologically a profound truth.

But let's get going.

In chapter1 we have seen that man is 'by nature' closer to the chimpanzee and gorilla than to the lion and the tiger.

Man is by nature (digestive tract, teeth) not a carnivore. Our psyche, too, has little of the characteristics of that of a carnivore, as Diamond and Diamond amusingly illustrate in their bestseller *Fit for Life*:

"We are as humans not even psychologically equipped to eat meat. Have you ever wandered around lush woodland while you filled your lungs with the pure air and listened *to singing of the birds?* Maybe it was after a rain shower and everything was clean and fresh. Sunlight filtered through the trees and sparkled in the moisture on the flowers and the grass. Maybe a striped squirrel happened to be on your path. What was your very first *instinctive impulse* at the sight of that little animal before you even had time to reflect? Did you shoot down on it like a hawk to grasp the little animal with your teeth, rip it apart and devour it, after which you choke down everything, flesh, blood, gut, skin and bones? Did you then lick off your lips contentedly and praise the Gods that you happened to choose this particular path on this very day so you got the opportunity to devour this delicious snack? Or would you instead, at the sight of the furry little animal have exclaimed tenderly, "Oh, what a sweet striped squirrel!""

An absurd picture with a kernel of truth. As an aside: if you, per chance, would have sighted wild strawberries you would eagerly have polished off a handful, licking your lips!

While meat is healthy food for the lion, it is unhealthy for humans. This already follows from the finding that regular consumption of red meat increases mortality risk, as we shall discuss below. But let me start with an introductory passage taken from my book *You can live longer,* published in 2000.

Before passing the disadvantages of meat in review, I would like to mention the outcome of a forced population experiment in Denmark. In the course of the First World War the Danes had virtually sold their whole livestock to the Germans and became almost vegetarians. During that period mortality decreased by 17 per cent. When in 1917 the Allies started a total blockade against Germany, the Danish people were also deprived of imported meat and their diet consisted mainly of (extra) potatoes and barley. One year after this forced semi-vegetarianism mortality from disease had dropped by 34 per cent. This mass-experiment gave the impetus to present-day epidemiology.

A study published in the *British Medical Journal* in 1994 showed that vegetarians had 40 per cent less cancers than non-vegetarians (omnivores). This fact on its own shows that a life-long meat diet is carcinogenic. A very important American study involving 88,000 women between 30-69 years showed that in those individuals who consumed red meat almost daily cancer incidence was 3.5 times higher than in women who ate little or no meat.

Professor Walter Willett of Harvard who headed the study gave the following comment in the New York Times, "If you stand back and look at the data, then the optimal amount of red meat should be zero."

In other words: just for this reason alone, you should, if you are sensible, stop eating red meat!

Of perhaps even greater significance is the finding in a Harvard study involving 38,000 subjects over a 28-year period that appeared in *The Archives of Internal Medicine,* that a daily portion red meat (the size of your hand palm) increased mortality risk with 13 per cent. Let me mention in passing that the study found that the risk of fatal heart disease increased by 18 per cent and cancer risk by 10 per cent.

With regard to conserved meat the risk percentage is even higher. The authors stated, "We found that a higher intake of red meat was associated with a significantly elevated risk of total, cardiovascular and cancer mortality."

The 'vitalist', the person who aspires to live a long healthy life and loves red meat is well advised to restrict the T-bone steak to once a week (on Friday?). This offers the double advantage that he/she can substantially restrict the consumption of baked and broiled food (see chapter 7), for who loves to eat a cooked beefsteak?

And the grilled T-bone steak of course carries its own risks (burnt meat, cancer risk).

One thing is clear: red meat should play only a minor role in the Paleo anti-aging diet. The Paleo diet is for those who *eat to live* and totally unsuitable for those who *live to eat*.

The essence of the Paleo anti-aging diet
Its essential features are:

1) no grains
2) little red meat
3) vegetables and fruit
4) beans, mushrooms and nuts

ad 1) The ban on the use of grains is in agreement with the evolutionary argument that the human organism is adapted to the diet prior to the agrarian revolution some 10,000 years ago but the reason for this ban in the anti-aging diet is that the starch in grains (the carbohydrates) are quickly converted to free glucose in the gut. The relatively high glycaemic index (peaks of blood glucose, see chapter 4) of grains, due to the quick conversion to free glucose, is harmful in the long run.

Rice and wheat are 'prohibited', which means that bread and pasta should be avoided. For the same reason potatoes are on the black list.

But every rule has its exception and here it is oatmeal. Oatmeal has a lower glycaemic index, 58, than other grains because of the presence of soluble fibre. Soluble fibre absorbs water in the gut and becomes viscous. Soluble fibre is slowly dissolved and releases the sugar content gradually.

Incidentally, it may be mentioned that bananas too have a low glycaemic index (50).

So, if you're used to eating bread in the morning, you would be well advised to substitute it by oatmeal (with soymilk rather than milk).

ad 2) As we have seen, the main reason for eating little red meat is that it shortens lifespan.

ad 3) Numerous scientific studies have shown an inverse relationship between the consumption of fresh vegetables and fruit and chronic disorders. The more you consume it the lower the chance of developing a chronic ailment. The *American Institute for Cancer Research* states: "Diets that contain a lot of vegetables and fruit prevent 20 per cent of cancer cases."

If you eat 200 grams of beefsteak there is little space left for vegetables. In a 3-star restaurant, but also in the typical American diet, the meat chunk comes first and vegetables come second or third.

In the anti-aging diet it is the other way round: vegetables first, the rest is secondary.

A personal example: my typical evening meal consists of carrots, broccoli, cauliflower, spinach and one boiled egg. Instead of potatoes I eat a bit of beans or peas or one potato (this as a concession to my taste buds). The taste is determined by the sauce of your choice. As an additional source of protein I use a whey protein powder drink.

I'll omit the discussion of fruit. Blackberries deserve special mention because of their high content of antioxidants and cancer-fighting nutrients. Avocado, a fruit with highly nutritious properties, deserves a place of honour in your delicious salads!

ad 4) All I would like to mention is that beans, by the presence of soluble fibre, have - like oatmeal – a low glycaemic index.

Very important advice
Since food (nutrition) is a very important and extensive theme and since only one chapter in this book is devoted to this subject, I highly recommend the excellent book of Kris Verburgh M.D., the Food Hourglass.

The views of Dr. Verburgh and mine on the role of diet in health and aging run parallel, as is illustrated by this quote on oatmeal from his book:

"Oatmeal porridge is made from oatmeal and is thus a grain product. Oatmeal porridge is the only grain product that is recommended in this book."

His book also offers recipes that may help you to turn the Paleo anti-aging diet into a feast!

He also states: "… potatoes, rice, and pasta you may replace by legumes (beans, peas, lentils, tofu), mushrooms and extra vegetables."

Order the Food Hourglass today at Amazon and you will be richly rewarded.

Let me end this chapter with a happy note: although milk, quark, etc. are discouraged, cheese and butter in moderate amounts are allowed.

Be flexible: compromise
Especially for the Paleo-diet the rule "cheating is allowed" holds.

Even the most fervent supporter of this diet, the Swedish physician–researcher Staffan Lindeberg, author of the authoritative book on the Paleo-diet *Food and Western Disease* 'cheats'. He writes, *"Very few people are able to follow this kind of dietary advice without compromises (I cannot manage this, for example)."*

So, he too 'cheats', i.e. does not adhere strictly to the diet.

'Cheating', 'sinning' is allowed, no 'sinning' is a *must*. One day you will be lying on your deathbed and realize you have never sinned. What regrets! But then it is too late ...

Stew (high glycaemic index) and a Magnum (very bad) are allowed occasionally. A slice of bread with cheese and butter is fine, as is an occasional barbecue. And do visit your favourite restaurant in Chinatown and help yourself to a lot of white rice and Chinese noodles.

The Mediterranean diet: second best

Although the so-called Mediterranean diet is recommended since the fifties as the healthiest Western diet the definitive proof was still missing: a well-designed statistical study.

In February 2012 the results of a 5-year randomized study involving 7,000 subjects were published on the website of the *New England Journal of Medicine*.

About 30 per cent of heart attacks, strokes and death from a heart condition can be prevented in high risk individuals (diabetes, smoking, high blood pressure) when they switch to the Mediterranean diet rich in fish, fruit, vegetables, beans, nuts and olive oil.

It is worth mentioning that all researchers (18) switched to the Mediterranean diet after the study was completed.

By the way, you may well have noticed that the Mediterranean diet has a lot in common with the Paleo-anti-aging diet. Wow, what a liberating thought ...

Chapter 3

How much protein a day?

This is a brief chapter on a complex subject. Just as with vitamins there are tables developed by the national health services and the WHO, that tell us how many grams of protein we must consume daily in order to stay healthy. How is such a table constructed?

For its construction the so-called *sodium balance method* is used (don't get alarmed!).

Proteins are made up of the atoms (building blocks) hydrogen (H), oxygen (O), carbon (C) and nitrogen (N). In our body synthesis break-down of our body proteins constantly takes place and these break-down products partially leave the body via the urine, faeces, etc.

Via the urine the 'protein waste' is secreted as urea.

If we want to know how much protein is needed daily we have to measure the amount of protein lost to the outside world. As measure nitrogen (N) lost in urine, faeces, and even the breath (ammonia) is used. When this value is multiplied by a certain factor (6.25), the amount of protein lost is determined.

Suppose this is 50 gram a day, then 50 gram daily from food is needed to insure that the body is not 'in the red'.

To establish how much body protein is lost daily, test persons are put on a protein-free diet and the loss of nitrogen in urine, faeces, skin and respiration is measured.

Putting all sources of protein loss together the following list is obtained (N in mg per kg body weight):

via urine	37
via faeces	12
via skin	3
via sperm	2
total	54

The total loss of protein per kilogram body weight is obtained by multiplying this result with 6.25, 6.25x54=337.5 (rounded off to 0.34 gram.)

The loss of 0.34 gram protein per kg body weight must be compensated by food intake. This means that the minimum daily protein requirement for an adult (male in this example) is 0.34 gram per kg body weight.

According to the official tables the daily protein requirement is considerably higher than we have found. Why is this? Well, 0.34 is the average value of the test persons studied, and just as you have tall and small persons, there is a spread in the individual values of the (minimal) protein requirement.

In order to make sure that the protein need of 98 per cent of the population is covered, statisticians have added 30 per cent to this value, so that in the official table the minimum value becomes 0.45 gram protein per kg body weight, instead of 0.34.

But with all this computation we ain't there yet! Forget it, for researchers are a bunch of oddballs. They want to make everything, including man, watertight. However I won't bother you any further with their arguments. Initially the factor 0.45 is increased to 0.57 to end at 0.79 gram protein per kilogram body weight a day (rounded off to 0.80) for young adults. So it is more than twice the initial experimentally determined value of 0.34.

This value, 0.80 gr/kg is the American RDA-value (Recommended Daily Allowance).

The RDA value proposed by the WHO is considerably lower, however,: 0.50 gr/kg.

My advice is that in daily practice your protein intake may lie between 0.35 gr/kg and 0.80.

If your weight is – like mine - 70 kg, you would need 0.35x 70 = 24.5, or, rounded off, 25 gr protein/day. You don't need to worry about too little protein, simply because the body quickly adapts its nitrogen balance to the protein intake (see frame).

In the West no-one has ever died from lack of protein (except some people in old people's homes who often skip meals because they taste awful). Many, however, are dying every day from protein overload, which is harmful for the kidneys (especially meat protein) and the bones (osteoporosis with its consequences).

> The adaptability of the body to different levels of protein consumption is clearly shown by the following experiment. The test person (a woman, weighing 58 kg) was first put on a protein–rich diet (25 gr nitrogen). Then she was suddenly switched to a protein–poor diet (17 gr nitrogen). The first two days the nitrogen balance was negative (-2 gr nitrogen). Then the balance oscillated between zero and slightly positive. In other words, within 3 days the body had fully adapted to the protein-poor diet, in the sense that the body had lowered its own protein breakdown to the same degree.
>
> This and similar studies offer the precise proof that our body easily adapts to a diet relatively low in protein. The vegetarian who eats a varied diet should never worry about "too little protein".

To give you an idea how easy it is for a vegetarian to meet his protein need, I offer the following example:

1 portion broccoli	6.50 g
1 portion peas	8.40 g
1 portion yoghurt	5.40 gr
white of 3 eggs	4.50 gr
1 portion rice	3.75 gr
3 slices brown bread	6.75 gr
total	35.30 gr protein

So, ample for your daily protein requirements.

Suggestion: If you want more protein than you suspect your diet contains, you can supplement it with a protein powder as a soya milk drink.

Well-known products are Protifar (Nutricia) and Whey Protein (Solgar). Since I eat frugally I use a protein drink containing 20 gr gram protein daily for extra insurance, given the fact that no-one knows my 'optimal' value, except that it lies somewhere in the range mentioned. Incidentally, I have no problem with the drink, as I use it to swallow my nutrient supplements (chapter **38**).

Chapter 4

Sugar: the White Death

Sugar is bad, we all know this. On the internet you'll find numerous websites that mention more than a hundred harmful effects of sugar: from tooth decay to cancer.

Here I shall restrict myself to some major points, of which *glycation* and *insulin stimulation* are the most important.

Are you too addicted to 'sweet'? As I mentioned I eat my oatmeal for breakfast, and apart from a sweetener I cannot resist adding a tablespoon of Honey. Sugar (sucrose) is both bad and dangerous, which doesn't mean that you should not transgress occasionally with ice cream, a cake or even a coke.

Culturally, sugar has a good reputation, fat(s) a bad one, but sugar is far more harmful than solid fats.

Sugar is deeply engrained in our culture and collective psyche. Ray Kurzweil in his anti-aging book offers a striking example. "How ya doin', sugar?" and "Honey, I'm home." You don't say to your loved one – although fat is far less harmful than sugar, "How ya doin', fatso, or, "Lardy, I'm home."

Why is sugar so harmful ?
Because sugar increases the insulin level and insulin is a risk factor for heart infarction and stroke. Canadian researchers Despres and LaMarche state that a permanently elevated insulin blood level (so-called insulinaemia) is the second main factor for cardiac infarction. The optimum insulin value is 12 mU/l or lower. An insulin value above 30 doubles the risk of a heart attack, while values above 37 triple the risk. In the long run a high insulin level exerts a corrosive effect on the blood vessels and the heart. The adverse action of too much sugar also follows from the classic study of Yudlin, who compared the sugar consumption of 65 patients who

had suffered a heart attack with that of the control group. The sugar consumption of the cardiac patients was on the average 170 pounds/year and that of the control group 80. Statistically it could be shown with a confidence level of 99.999 per cent that excessive sugar consumption was the cause of the heart attack.

Historically too - from the beginning of the 20th century – the enormous increase in the incidence of heart attacks correlated with the explosive increase of sugar consumption (and, this is worth noting, not with the consumption of fats or saturated fats). When the Nestor of American cardiology, Professor Paul Dudley White (president Eisenhower's cardiologist) began his career in 1920 heart infarction was a medical curiosity and the sugar consumption in the USA relatively low.[4]

Most persuasive is the observation of the researcher M. Cohen, who found that among recently emigrated Jews from Yemen (less than 10 years ago) heart diseases were rare, despite the fact that their diet in Yemen was rich in animal fat (but poor in sugar). The Yemenite Jews who had lived in Israel for more than 25 years had a high incidence of heart infarction, corresponding to the high sugar consumption in Israel.

But isn't heart infarction closely associated with animal fats, I can hear you think.

If that is true, then a high incidence of heart disease should be found among the Masai and Samburu nomadic tribes in Eat-Africa, who subsist exclusively on milk, beef and mutton. They have little heart disease and heart infarction is rare.

Glycaemic index
De glycaemic index or GI is a (crude) measure of the effect of carbohydrates (sugars and starches: yes, technically sugar is also a carbohydrate) of the rise of the blood sugar level after a meal.

Glucose has the strongest effect and has – by definition – a GI value of 100.

Foods with GI values above 70 (white bread, white rice, cornflakes, glucose, breakfast cereals) are harmful, while GI values below 55 (fruits, vegetables, leguminous plants, full grains, nuts) are 'safe'.

---

4   The low incidence of heart attacks in the twenties could also be due to 'missed diagnoses', since cardiology only took off in the thirties, after the invention of the electrocardiogram

> The GI value is not the whole story: eating 10 gram of a food with a high GI value is less harmful than eating 100 gram of a food with a lower. So quantity matters.
>
> **Sugars and carbohydrates**
> Glucose and fructose are the simplest sugars and are (thus) called mono-saccharides (mono=1). sugar or sucrose, is a chemical compound made up of glucose and fructose and is called a di-saccharide (di=2)
> Starch consists of strings of glucose molecules and is referred to as a poly-saccharide (poly=many)
> When you eat starch it is converted by enzymes into glucose, but since the uptake occurs slowly, de blood sugar rise after a meal is less steep and high than when you consume the 'fast-acting' glucose. Hence the lower GI value of starch.
>
> **Note**
> Although fructose has a low GI value it is not harmless. Excessive consumption of fructose has little effect on the blood glucose level but increases the blood cholesterol level, as fructose is converted into acetate in the liver, which is partially converted into cholesterol.

Sugar and too much starch are dangerous because over time they elevate the glucose level 'jerkily' and with that also the average insulin level. The dangers of too much insulin are fully discussed elsewhere in this book. Here I just want to mention that a carbohydrate-rich diet leads to overweight by increasing the insulin level.

Have a cup of coffee (without sugar, a sweetener is all right) and I'll explain everything in simple terms.

All cells, such as muscles and the heart – that use fats as a source of energy, or cells that store fat (fat cells), have an enzyme called LPL (lipoprotein lipase).

LPL is referred to as the gatekeeper of the fat cells. The more active LPL the more fat is taken up by the fat cells. Which hormone regulates the activity of the gatekeeper?

Insulin. The more insulin, the more active LPL, so the more fat the gatekeeper pushes into the bulging fat cell![5]

---

[5] In fat tissue insulin increases the LPL activity, in muscles it decreases its activity. When insulin is secreted, fat is stored in fat tissue and the muscles must switch to glucose for energy. When the insulin level decreases, the LPL activity in the fat cells declines and the LPL activity in the muscle cells increases - the fat cells release fatty acids and the muscles take them up as fuel.

The result? Overweight or at least a beer belly!

It is of some interest to mention the personal experience of Ray Kurzweil, author of the life-extension bestseller *Fantastic Voyage* and one of the smartest guys on this planet. Let me quote:

"At 35 I developed diabetes type 2. My doctor prescribed the conventional treatment with insulin, but this made de situation worse by causing a considerable degree of weight gain. That in its turn resulted in an apparent need for more insulin. "(unquote).

With Ray the injected insulin caused weight gain, while with a carbohydrate-rich diet the elevated blood sugar level makes you fat via the secretion of extra insulin. In both cases insulin is the villain!

As we shall discuss later fat intake is not the cause of obesity, but carbohydrates (including sugar). This explains why the carbohydrate-poor Atkins diet and the South Beach diet (low GI-index foods) are so effective in slimming.

Another danger of sugar (and too much carbs) is the so-called saccharification (also called 'caramelization'), or, using the technical term, glycation.

Glycation
It is sometimes said that as you grow older you turn sour. This is wrong. You become sweeter.

This is due to the 'caramelization 'of proteins, a normal phenomenon that is called 'glycation'. Sugar is very 'sticky' and the higher the glucose level, the more glucose attaches to proteins, whereby these become 'denatured'.

This 'caramelization' is used in a test to assess the severity of diabetes. It is – don't be alarmed - the HbA1c test. With this test the percentage of the haemoglobin (Hb) affected by glucose is measured. A value of 7 % or higher is considered abnormal and indicates diabetes. People without diabetes also have caramelized Hb, with values between 4.5 - 5.5 per cent.

The rule is: the higher your blood sugar level, the higher the percentage caramelized haemoglobin.

The reason that in the long run not all of our haemoglobin is caramelized and thus damaged, is that red blood cells only have e lifespan of some 120 days. So, there is constant renewal of haemoglobin.

This is just an example to show that 'caramelization' just like' aging' is an on-going process. At this very moment, in all your tissues, the sugar that supplies your body with energy is also caramelizing your body, exactly the same process (at lower temperature) that gives onions, peanuts and the turkey in the oven their nutty flavour and brown colour. Caramelizing proteins means 'denaturing' proteins, change their molecule's three-dimensional structure and thereby inactivating them. These caramelized proteins have a special name – don't be put off - Advanced Glycation products (AGEs). As Wiki says: "It is a collective term for proteins that are irreparably damaged, because sugar groups (like glucose) are attached to them and the protein is degraded."

The harmful effects of glycation and its end products AGEs often only become manifest at later stages, such as 'old age spots' and cataract, characterized by brown spots in the lens, whereby the transparent crystalline proteins get clouded. Not 'in the light of day' but very much present, are other consequences of AGEs, such as cross-linking, a process whereby protein molecules attach to one another and tissues, like the arterial wall, become rigid and inelastic. Here the result is elevated (systolic) blood pressure.

Cross-linking is the same process that turns old newspaper yellow and makes the tires of your car and screen wipers brittle.

Yes, if you're not careful growing old is no picnic; both on the outside and on the inside you become as crusty as a burned beefsteak, the product of caramelization.

In which group of people we see the most serious consequences of glycation? In diabetes patients, which is the direct proof of the thesis, "The higher the blood sugar level, the more glycation and

AGEs. Conversely, the lower the glucose level the less glycation."

This is besides keeping the glucose level low for keeping the insulin level low another reason to keep your glucose level low with a low-calorie diet low in sugar and carbohydrates (bread).

Diabetes is aging magnified

Diabetes is nothing but 'accelerated aging'. Almost all 'complications' of diabetes are due to glycation or too much insulin.

Diabetes is the most common cause of kidney failure (1/3 of dialysis patients are diabetics) and the severity of kidney disease in diabetes is determined by the level of kidney-AGEs (glycation end product), that crosslink the proteins and thus makes them less permeable.

In humans researchers have found that also within the 'normal' range (no diabetes) higher blood glucose values are associated with more glycation damage and higher mortality.

People with diabetes live on the average 7-8 years shorter. Since the disease usually occurs mostly after fifty, this means that the average diabetes patient (type 2) has a remaining life expectancy that is 20 to 30 per cent lower than the average life expectancy.

But since maturity-onset diabetes is only a blow-up of 'normal' aging by glycation (where there is glucose, there is glycation!), it implies that we can increase our life expectancy by keeping our glucose level as low as possible.

We shouldn't be satisfied with staying within the 'normal range', but make sure that our glucose level is at the lower end or even below the 'normal range'.

I would like to end this section with a quote from the authoritative book *Life Extension Revolution* by Philip Miller, M.D., a publication from the Life Extension Foundation that spends millions of dollars yearly on supporting basic research on 'life extension' and aging.

"In many respects the progression of diabetes is in fact a picture of accelerated aging. And both in diabetes as in aging glycation is responsible for much of the damage to the organs and tissues. Remember that glyction is caused by the sugar in your blood. Glycation is a problem for everyone, not only for the diabetes patient."

Practical lesson:
Avoid as much as possible sweets: sugar, pastries, dessert, but also soft drinks and be 'abstemious' with carbohydrates like bread, pasta, potatoes, etc.

Chapter 5

Metformin: the 'youth pill'

The purpose of this book is to point the way to 1) staying youthful longer, 2) to extend your lifespan and 3) to decrease your risk of cancer.

This is very important as cancer is closely linked to greying of the population and increases dramatically after 60. To give you an idea: when you are 80 your chances of getting cancer are 2000 times greater than when you were 20. And remember 1 in 3 gets cancer in his lifetime.

What you have to do to implement all this can be written on a A4 page and if you would accept my authority you would immediately start the program and ..., stop just as quickly. Why? Because you are only really motivated to do what is required if you truly understand the underlying scientific reasons for it.

So it will be necessary to take you on a quest in *terra incognita* (unknown territory): the function(s) of your body and body cells. Difficult material? Fortunately not really, for – as the Nobel Prize winner, the physicist professor Rutherford often said, "Good science, however complex, you should be able to explain to your barkeeper." *Skål!* To your health.

Let's get started ...

Metformin: the 'youth pill'
Metformin, a substance derived from the French lily, has been used since the seventies to lower the blood sugar level in diabetes. So it is an anti-diabetic drug and the one that is most often prescribed. I use it myself since a couple of years and have no diabetes. Because Metformin also lowers the blood sugar level in non-diabetics and

hardly has any side effects. Moreover it offers, as studies in humans have shown, an important protection against cancer, the sword of Damocles hanging over the head of the aging individual.

But now the question immediately arises in your mind, "Why is it important to keep glucose- and insulin levels low if you want to slow down aging and extend lifespan? Is this just 'theory' or has it been experimentally proven? This is the theme of the next section.

Calorie restriction

Since the classic studies by Dr. Clive McCay in the thirties thousands of studies have been done all over the world on test animals, varying from the mouse to dogs, whereby the test animals since early youth receive 30 per cent less calories than normal. The result?

In nearly all cases the maximal age of the test animals rose by 30 per cent, while the animals remained relatively young and healthy in old age. Even when calorie restriction was applied in middle-age or later the aging process was strongly retarded while the test animals lived longer than normal. In human terms this would mean that humans on such a diet could reach a maximal age of 160 instead of the current 120.

One thing is crystal clear: extreme calorie reduction, even when started late, is the golden path to 'youth conservation' and a longer life.

But no-one – certainly not you or me – can stick to such a diet for more than a week. For this reason scientists wanted to know by what bio-chemical mechanism calorie restriction exerts its magical effects, in the hope of finding a drug that would exert the same effects without dietary restrictions.

The solution proved simple: calorie restriction works by keeping the glucose level and the insulin level low.

Can it be simpler?

For the layman too, it appears obvious that calorie restriction keeps the blood sugar level low, just like overeating increases the glucose level (resulting in so-called pre-diabetes).

The next question raised was of course: is there a safe drug available that can mimic this effect: a low sugar level and a low insulin level?

How would you tackle the problem? Inject insulin? Yes, then the glucose level drops, but the insulin level rises. Less carbohydrates and/or calorie restriction? Yes, but you will only get the anti-aging effect when you eat 30 per cent less, although sugar and calorie restriction is of course always a good thing. You could also reduce the absorption of sugar and carbohydrates in the gut by using substances like L-arabinose, but this is not sufficiently effective.

No, the best way is to put the brake on the release of glucose manufactured in the liver into the bloodstream.

Just as the liver produces cholesterol and releases it into the bloodstream (this explains why you always have cholesterol in your blood even if you are a vegan), so the liver produces glucose. In fact the liver manufactures a kind of starch, glycogen that is stored in the liver as an energy source. When as a result of lack of food the blood glucose level drops critically then the liver swings into action: glucose is set free from glycogen and is released into the bloodstream. In the evolutionary sense a brilliant mechanism. In modern man this emergency-mechanism has become disordered: the liver continues to release glucose to the bloodstream despite sufficient supply of glucose from food.

Our glucose content in the blood - both of us having normal glucose values I trust - is thus the result of two sources: the glucose supply from food and the glucose release from the liver. Scientists have found the best way to mimic calorie-restriction is to cut off or reduce the glucose release from the liver. This leads to a drastic lowering of the blood glucose level in the order of 25 per cent).

As a consequence of this low glucose concentration the insulin level is low too. Although the low insulin is here just the result of low glucose the main thing for the anti-aging 'imitation' of calorie restriction is the low insulin level.[6]

Metformin lowers the glucose blood level and thus the insulin level by slowing down the release of glucose by the liver.[7]

The following passage is taken from the book THE LIFE EXTENSION REVOLUTION, a publication of the Life Extension Foundation (USA), the leading non-profit organisation on life-extension.

"The most promising results so far have been obtained with metformin (trade name Glucophage) that was originally developed for diabetes. Besides its ability to increase the insulin sensitivity of the tissues and lower the glucose– and insulin levels, metformin diminishes appetite, body weight and body fat both in diabetics and non-diabetics. It also protects against glycation and its harmful effects. Many scientists recommend the use of metformin for the whole population."

The book appeared in 2005; since then the effectiveness of calorie restriction mimetics ('imitators') like metformin have been convincingly shown experimentally.

As I mentioned earlier calorie restriction extends the maximal lifespan of most species by about 30 per cent (with exceptions, like the rhesus monkey) when the hunger diet is started early.

The golden standard for life extension is the increase in maximal lifespan (120 years for man), not the mean lifespan (life expectancy). This has little meaning within this context, as is already clear from the use of antibiotics that have increased mean lifespan in human populations.

In human terms, if you wish your sweet little boy a long and healthy life then you should put him on a permanent vita-

---

6   Insufficient insulin production by sick or deficient pancreas cells, like in diabetes, is not the solution, since it leads to a sharp increase in the glucose level.

7   Metformin activates the enzyme AMPK in the liver, which cuts back both the synthesis and secretion of glucose and so lowers the glucose blood level.

min-rich hunger diet with plenty of spinach and he will live to celebrate his 160th birthday! It is that simple. You yourself had better take a CR-mimetic (CR= calorie restriction) like metformin to replicate the effects of 'hunger' and thus achieve the same results.

Scientists have discovered a number of CR-mimetics, and in 2009 three independent groups under the auspices of the National Institute of Aging (USA), have given a mimetic to mice only at a more advanced age (equivalent to 60 years in humans) in order to find out whether this daily treatment would be able, just like calorie restriction, to extend *maximal* lifespan. The results were positive, as we will discuss below.

Allow me to digress a bit. Incidentally, metformin is one of the mimetics that extend maximal life span in mice, but in these tests the drug was started at an early age which makes it less relevant to the aging individual.

Let me mention one example In 2008 Anisimov's group in Saint Petersburg found that in mice metformin increased maximal life span by 10 per cent and the mean (average) life span by 38 per cent.[8]

Let's return to the afore-mentioned studies.

The average extension of the maximal age of mice whom had been given the CR-mimetic rapamycin from middle age on was 12 per cent as compared to that of untreated mice.

(Here the "maximal life span" is defined as the average length of life of the oldest 10 per cent of the population.)

This is a spectacular result!

Theoretically it would mean that the maximal life span of man (120 years) would be about 135 if everybody would be on CR-mimetics like rapamycin or metformin!

Even more amazing is that the mean lifespan increased by more than a third. Since the life expectancy in – say- the Netherlands

---

[8] Anisimov, V.N. et al "Metformin slows aging and extends lifespan of female SHR mice,", Cell Cycler, 7, 2769, 2008.

is about 80 years, this would theoretically suggest that the life expectancy would be 107 years if the whole population would be on rapamycin!

Regrettably rapamycine has too many unpleasant side effects for human use.

Metformin works however in the same way, is just as powerful and has no serious side effects. Currently a study comparing the life extension effects of rapamycin and metformin is being conducted but the results will not be in before 2015 (Current date: 2013).

On the basis of the existing animal studies with metformin and its known action as a CR-mimetic metformin is recommended by scientists as the ideal drug to increase the 'number of 'healthy years' in the elderly, to slow down the aging process and to increase life span.

The recommended dose is 500 mg metformin taken twice daily.

> **How do I obtain metformin?**
> Metformin is only available on prescription. The recommended dose for anti-aging is, as mentioned, 500mg twice daily.
>
> The diligent searcher may be able to find a website where it can be obtained without prescription.
>
> Just like aspirin that was originally prescribed as an analgesic (anti-pain drug) currently also to protect against thrombosis and colon cancer, so metformin is prescribed by many health-conscious doctors as protection against cancer and as anti-aging drug.
>
> If you're a diabetic and you are already taking for your blood sugar say 2 tablets metformin (500mg), you can safely double this dose for use as an anti-aging tablet without running the risk of hypoglycaemia. Of course you would have to discuss this fully with your physician and obtain his blessing!
>
> As a non-diabetic you could ask your physician for a prescription telling him about the anti-aging benefits of metformin. You could also tell him that you wish to further lower your 'normal' glucose level (which may well be on the high side of normal) with metformin as a preventive measure against developing the condition called pre-diabetes (1 in 5 people have pre-diabetes).
>
> It is important to some extra vitamin B12 if you are on metformin (at least 50 mcg orally daily) because metformin may interfere with the absorption of vitamin B12, which in the long run may lead to neuropathy, a painful condition which may also be caused by the high glucose found in diabetes.

> Since in rare cases metformin may cause fatal lactic acid poisoning in patients suffering from kidney failure (most of them diabetics) it is formally recommended to undergo a kidney function test before starting on metformin. In my opinion this is advisable when you are a diabetic. For non-diabetics without kidney problems such a test is deemed unnecessary on the basis of the extremely low risk involved (less than one in 5 million).

A very important additional benefit is that metformin reduces the risk of getting cancer by about 50 per cent. This aspect will be fully discussed in chapter 7.

Medical Appendix

Since rapamycin provided the experimental proof that CR-mimetics can extend maximal life span and slow down aging it is of interest to mention the historical origin of this drug and its mode of action.

Rapamycin was discovered in 1964 in the mud of Easter Island in the Pacific Ocean, famous for its mysterious sculptures of huge human heads. Rapamycine (Rapa, the name of the volcanic island Rapa Nui) is a defensive substance produced by a bacterium living in the mud. This compound possesses a number of magical properties and is widely used against tissue rejection in organ transplants because of its inhibition of immune cell proliferation. Scientists became intrigued by the finding that Rapamycin was found to inhibit both the proliferation of yeast cells and mammalian cells. This shows that the compound suppresses the action of a growth-regulating gene that has been conserved during the billion years of evolution (Cells grow, increase in size as they get ready to divide and proliferate). In 1991 this gene was identified in yeast. Three years later Stuart Schreiber of Harvard discovered the human gene, that was called the TOR-gen (Target of Rapamycine). This gene codes for the TOR enzyme that in the cell represents the spider in the web that regulates a complex of growth activities within the cell.
    TOR (gene and enzyme) turn out to possess a number of amazing properties.

TOR is a food sensor. When there is plenty of food TOR's activity increases, whereby the cells increase in size and start dividing. When food is scarce, TOR activity decreases sharply resulting in a sharp fall or cessation of cell growth (both cell volume and proliferation). Also, autophagy increases, the process that takes place in the lysosomes where cell breakdown products are recycled to new building blocks and fuel. When sufficient food is again available, TOR becomes more active again and autophagy decreases.

In connection with metformin (that keeps insulin low) the fact that the "signalling pathways" of TOR and insulin are closely interrelated is of crucial significance. Signalling pathways are series of molecular interactions that regulate the cell activities.

It is generally known that insulin is the hormone secreted by the pancreas during and after a meal that tells muscle cells and other cells to take up glucose from the blood. Glucose insensitivity means that the cells do not 'listen' sufficiently to this signal with the result that glucose accumulates in the bloodstream: diabetes. Less familiar is insulin's second function: it is a growth factor.

Insulin activates TOR as a result of which in the whole body cells start growing and proliferating. As mentioned earlier we know since the classic experiments of Clive MacCay in the thirties, that young test animals on a permanent hunger diet (calorie restriction) grow very slowly and live much longer.

In 1990 scientists found that "starved" cells in vitro curtail their growth by decreasing TOR-activity.

Here then is the link between TOR and aging: the lower TOR–activity, the slower cell growth and thus the slower aging of the cell (and the whole organism).[9]

---

[9] Incidentally it may be mentioned that a negative feedback exists between TOR and insulin pathways. The more TOR is stimulated the less responsive cells become to insulin. So they take up less glucose whereby the glucose blood level increases → more insulin secretion → more TOR stimulation → cells even less sensitive to insulin signals → further increase of blood glucose and insulin, etc. A vicious circle is established. The result is diabetes, accelerated aging and its 'symptoms': geriatric diseases. The basic cause is long-term over-eating.

Chapter 6

Overweight and cancer

Everybody knows that overweight is bad for you. It increases the risk of heart disease, diabetes, etc. Less well-known, however, is that overweight greatly increases the risk of getting cancer and that cancer in overweight people has a worse outcome. What is the probability that you're too heavy? Statistically speaking more than 50 per cent! In the USA 68 per cent of adults are overweight,

Cancer is the black hole on the path of your life. It is a matter of 'bad luck', it is a consequence of getting old and you can do nothing about it. "Oh, yea, don't smoke, don't get too much sun, eat healthy food and pray," one sighs, resigned to the slings and arrows of outrageous fortune.

When you are 81 your cancer risk is 2000 times greater than when you were 18. Yes, 2000 times! To put it into perspective: if you smoke your risk of getting lung cancer is 40 times greater than otherwise. So, 2000 is a lot. And this figure holds for people who are not overweight. With overweight you double the risk, so an overweight 81-old person has 4000 times the risk when he was 18.

Considering the fact that one in three persons gets cancer during his lifetime you may well want to reduce your cancer risk as much as possible.

A recent report of the American Institute of Cancer Research (AICR) states the excess body weight is now considered the major cause of cancer and calculates that in the USA overweight is responsible for 100 new cancer cases each year. Excess weight is the ideal breeding ground for cancer. The oncologist (cancer specialist) professor Michael Pollak of McGill University in Montreal, states, "Cancer loves the metabolic environment of the obese person."[10]

---

10 See also for example, F. Biancini, Overweight, obesity and cancer risk, The Lancet Oncology, 3, 565, 2002.

But before proceeding: what is too heavy?

The highest 'admissible' weight (kg) is your height (cm) minus 100. So, if you're 180 cm tall, you may weigh 80 kg at most. From the point of view of prevention it would be better if you weigh less. Apart from your weight your girth is of importance: when the waist-size (as measured across the navel) in the male is over 102 cm, or over 88cm in the female, then, using a colloquialism, a 'beer belly' is present, which, apart from body weight, entails some extra health risks, including diabetes, which by itself is a cancer risk factor.

Let me insert a personal note. I am 186 cm tall and for years my weight has been 86 kilo; I looked on the heavy side and definitely had an small 'beer belly'. Since a couple of years my weight has gone down to 72 kilo, complete with a flat stomach. Some people consider me too thin, but medically (and cosmetically) speaking I am quite pleased and below you'll learn why.

The calorie–cancer connection

Cancer researchers have not directly established a connection between cancer and overweight, but hit upon the idea that there should be a connection between cancer and overweight from animal experiments with underfeeding (calorie restriction, see also chapter 5). Cancer in animals is sharply decreased or prevented if animals are near-starved. Implanted (human) tumours grow much more slowly or do not develop at all. This was established for the first time by professor Peyton Rous (Nobel laureate) and was confirmed by Albert Tannenbaum, a pathologist from Chicago in 1942, who showed that rats on a hunger diet that kept them barely alive lived much longer, mainly from the prevention of cancer (the main cause of death in the species used). Incidentally it may be mentioned that a decrease in cancer incidence (occurrence) was also found in rhesus monkeys kept on a moderately restricted diet. Just as in chapter 5 the question asked here was, "Through what (biochemical) mechanism does calorie restriction act on the reduction of the number of cancer cases and on tumour growth?"

Here too the answer turned out to be: "Via a low insulin level."[11]

As early as 1960 scientists showed that insulin (and a hormone related to insulin, IGF) accelerates the growth and proliferation of both normal cells and cancer cells.

Insulin and IGF are, in higher concentration, cancer promoters. Insulin and IGF nourish cancer cells and are even able to turn a normal cell into a cancer cell.

Would you like to know how insulin acts on a cell and how it may eventually cause cancer? Then listen to an amazing tale.

All our normal cells use oxygen to produce energy.

Cancer cells however are able to produce energy without oxygen, i.e. by a primitive and inefficient process that is similar to the energy production in bacteria. The fuel is glucose. Cancer cells produce one tenth of the energy (per glucose molecule) produced by normal cells. This oxygen-free process is called 'glycolysis', whereby instead of carbon dioxide (CO_2) lactic acid is formed as a by-product.

Thus the cancer cell is very inefficient and requires 10 times more fuel (glucose) than A NORMAL CELL.

The cancer cell devours glucose, resulting in too little remaining for the body cells, resulting in the patient getting thinner: in medical jargon this is called "cachexia", an ominous symptom occurring in the final stages of the disease.

By the way the enormous combustion of glucose supplies within the cancer cell forms the basis of the PET scan for the diagnosis of cancer.[12]

What is the role of (too much) insulin in this process?

The more insulin in the bloodstream the more glucose enters the cell. With too much insulin in the blood (so-called hyper-insulinaemia) like in obesity, there is a risk that the cell is flooded with glucose. The result? The energy production in the cell switches

---

[11] IGF too, plays a role, see medical appendix.
[12] PET = positron emission tomography, whereby fluorodeoxylglucose, a traceable analogue of glucose, is given to the patient.

over to the primitive process of glycolysis, the characteristic of the cancer cell. Since scientists who study the role of insulin in cancer agree that insulin supplies both the fuel (glucose) required for cancer cells to proliferate and the signals to sustain this process, the foundation is thus laid for the creation of a malignant tumour.[13]

That insulin can play a central role in the formation of cancer has been shown in various ways. Here I mention only one. We all possess certain genes that make sure that "cancer is suppressed". They are appropriately called 'suppressor genes'.

One of these suppressor genes is PTEN and it suppresses the action of the enzyme (don't get alarmed), bearing the difficult name P13 kinase. If there is a mutation that deactivates this gene P13 kinase becomes active. The result: cancer!

But P13 kinase can also be activated by a second factor: too much insulin.

With this the circle is closed but as an encore I'll mention the following:

When P13 kinase is activated, insulin becomes more effective in promoting the transport of glucose into the cell, as a result of which the process of glycolysis is further boosted and the fires of tumour growth are further fanned.

Cancer can thus be caused by the same mechanism (activation of P13 kinase) by both a mutation of the anticancer gene PTEN and by an excess of insulin, the hallmark of obesity.

It is clear that the lower the insulin level the safer, or in other words, the more protection against cancer.

Let me mention the following curious facts for those who are not yet fully convinced that "cancer loves insulin":

1. In order to grow cancer cells (e.g. breast cancer cells) in the lab one must always add insulin. If you leave out insulin the cancer cells die. "They are addicted to insulin," says Vuk Stambolic, a cancer researcher at the University of Toronto, Canada.

---

13   In the medical appendix this is further explained.

2. Many types of cancer (e.g. breast cancer, prostate cancer, colon cancer) possess, in contrast to most cell types in the body, insulin receptors in their membranes. These can be compared to locks in which the insulin key fits snugly. Muscle cells, liver cells, fat cells and three more types of cells among the 200 different body cells have insulin receptors. Breast cancer cells - to mention an example - are full of insulin receptors, while normal breast cells do not possess them.

This curbs the activity of digestive enzymes, resulting in the uptake of fewer calories. Its action is however weaker than that of metformin or rapamycin (See chapter 5).

Since an exhaustive discussion lies outside the scope of this book I will just mention a few possibilities from a scale of options.

1. orlistate: inhibits the enzyme lipase
2. acarbose: inhibits the enzyme alpha-glucodase
3. L-arabinose: inhibits the enzyme sucrose.

One could also use a natural appetite depressant, like the plant extract pinolenic acid that stimulates the secretion of appetite depressing hormones like chelocystokinin (CCK).

The Life Extension Foundation (USA) has developed the Calorie Restriction Mimetic Formula with the following composition (here presented only as an example):

Camelia sinensis	300 mg
quercittin	150 mg
trans-pterostilbenen	3 mg
trans-resveratrol	250 mg
proanthocyanids	50 mg

It is relevant within this context to mention two measures that may contribute to improving the course of the cancer process and prognosis by normalizing the combustion of glucose in the cancer cell. Although these two preparations exert their anti-cancer action via separate pathways, they have in common that they favourably influence the abnormal glucose metabolism (fermentation) in the cancer cell.

Complementary cancer treatment

1. **Avemar.** This is a plant extract that interferes with the Warburg effect and thereby induces the cancer cell to commit "suicide" (apoptosis). It is an 'over-the-counter' concentrated extract of fermented yeast germs and its effectiveness as a complementary therapy has been confirmed by more than a hundred published studies, of which more than 30 have appeared in leading science journals (e.g. Anticancer Res., 18, 2353, 1998. Avemar has no side effects and has the additional advantage that it maintains the white cell count during chemotherapy. A disadvantage is that it is expensive. For further information see e.g. www.avemarresearch.com and Google.

2. **Metformin.** Also in cancer in non-diabetics metformin lowers hyperinsulinaemia with about 23 per cent, which may contribute to its anti-cancer actions. Currently (2013) a large study under the auspices of the National Cancer Institute of Canada is under way to study the role of metformin as a complementary measure in cancer. Although this complementary action of metformin has not as yet been scientifically confirmed it is a rational choice for the cancer patient. As mentioned metformin inhibits the AKt activation and thereby exerts its anti-proliferative action.

3. **Dichloroacetate.** The then promising preparation DCA (dichloroacetate), which, like Avemar, works by interfering with the Warburg-effect ("fermentation") is no longer recommended because of the considerable risk of neuropathy (paralysis) .

Medical Appendix

According to the present understanding by leading cancer researchers the most common fundamental cause of cancer is the transformation of the healthy cell into a 'fermenting cell', a degenerate cell, which, like bacteria, produces energy via aerobic glycolysis (Warburg effect).

The Nobel Prize winner Svent Györgi proposed this theory in the seventies, which has now been experimentally substantiated.

The main causal factor in this transformation is abnormally high insulin levels. This activates the enzyme P13K, which accelerates the process. In minority of cancers a mutation of the tumour suppressor gene PTEN is the cause, as a result of which the action of P13K can take place unimpeded.

The transformation of such a "fermenting cell" into a cancer cell is usually the result of mutations from the massive productions of free radicals during (aerobic) glycolysis. The primary factor is the Warburg effect and the cancer cell is the secondary result of the Warburg effect. This theory was already formulated in the twenties by the Nobel Prize winner Otto Warburg, but completely ignored or played down by the cancer community. This lasted until the mid-eighties, when Lewis Cantley and his co-workers proved the central role of the enzyme P13 kinase in the development of most cancers. The rest is history ...

Notes

- The Warburg theory is 'old', the mutation theory is 'modern' and 'thus' correct, according to conventional wisdom. According to the official history the mutation theory was first advanced by C.O. Nordling in 1953 and precisely formulated by A.C. Knudson in 1971. But in fact the mutation theory is older than the Warburg theory and was proposed as early as 1928 by Karl Brauwer under the telling title "Mutationstheorie der Geschwulst-Entstehung".

- Although up till now more than 100 (proto) oncogenes and 30 tumour suppressor genes have been identified it is well established that the Warburg effect represents a necessary condition for the development of cancer. The aerobic glycolysis can be the result of a mutation in a proto-oncogene, hypoxia and other factors, including hyper-insulinaemia.

- In patients with diabetes type-2 on metformin the incidence of pancreas cancer is 60 per cent lower than in those patients treated with insulin or insulin inducing drugs, like sulvonylurea's.
Metformin exerts the following actions:

1. increased insulin sensitivity
2. increased glucose uptake by the cell
3. increased oxidation of fatty acids
4. decreased glucose absorption (in gut)
5. last but not least: decreased insulin level by blocking the glucose outflow from the liver (see above).

It is of interest that AMPK activation in P53-nullcells (like in many cancer types) induces apoptosis. Metformin activates AMPK, not only in the liver but also in cancer cells, just like phenformin.

- IGF, "insulin-like growth factor" has a chemical structure related to that of insulin. Its production (largely in the liver) is stimulated by growth hormone. It is of interest that cancer cells possess two to three times more IGF receptors than healthy cells, which makes them more sensitive for the IGF in their environment. In rodents the presence of functional IGF receptors is a necessary condition for cancer growth. Blockage of the IGF receptors leads to strong inhibition or suppression of cancer growth. In genetically modified mice with only ¼ the IGF blood level of normal mice tumour growth and metastasizing of transplanted human tumours is greatly reduced. When in these mice IGF is injected, tumour growth and metastasizing accelerate. This proves the activating role of IGF in cancer.

- Mutatis mutandis the same is found with insulin.

Chapter 7

Metformin and cancer prevention

This short chapter is intended for those readers who have skipped chapter 6 on de supposition that because of their normal weight it would not be applicable to them. If you're interested in cancer prevention I would urge you to read chapter 6 attentively. Here I will summarize the main points discussed in chapter 6.

Because cancer occurs infrequently in test animals on "calorie restriction" (30 per cent less calories than normal) and cancer incidence increases with body weight in both test animals and humans scientists have found that insulin is a major causal factor (Overweight is responsible for a quarter to one half of many cancers and "the list is growing" wrote Rudolf Kaaks in *Nature Reviews Cancer*).
The golden rule is,"the lower the glucose and insulin blood level the lower the cancer risk and conversely." High insulin values (so-called hyper insulinaemia) increase the risk of cancer.
In a sound bite you might say, "Cancer increases with age (geriatric disease) and with body weight."

But before proceeding I would like to mention the generally accepted measure of the 'ideal' body weight. This is called (don't be alarmed!) the BMI (body mass index), which is computed by a simple formula from your length (cm) and your weight (kg). You can have it computed by typing in Google 'compute BMI'. A value below 18.5 is 'too skinny' and values between 25 and 30 mean 'overweight'. Above 30 is truly 'obese'. My value used to be 24.8 for years. Fortunately it is down to 20.8 since a couple of years. Fortunately, for (within limits) 'the lower the better', unless it is the result of smoking, cocaine or an underlying condition.

Let us continue.

If the incidence (frequency) of cancer increases with body weight you would expect that cancer occurs less often in skinny people than in people of 'normal' weight? Is this true? No, but this tells us very little since a 'too low' body weight is often the result of harmful factors like smoking, poor nutrition, cocaine, cancer, or an underlying disease.

We have to look elsewhere: to Okinawa.

As you may possibly have heard the inhabitants of the Japanese island Okinawa have the highest life expectancy and the lowest cancer incidence in the world. To illustrate: Okinawans have 80 per cent less breast cancer and prostate cancer, 50 per cent less colon cancer etc. than in the rest of Japan and elsewhere.

The cancer incidence in Okinawa is very low as compared to the West and to the rest of Japan.

What is their 'secret'?

Their lifestyle, where the emphasis is on a low-calorie diet, less than 1500 calories a day for men instead of the 3000 calories per day that are consumed by Western men. Of course other factors such as a lot of physical exercise (heavy farm work even in old age), soy products, and lots of fish, a positive outlook, etc. are involved, but according to the experts the calorie restricted diet is the main factor.

Eat till you are 80 per cent full. The Okinawans call this rule: *Hara Hachi Bu* (stomach eighty per cent full). Leave the table when there is still space in your stomach, a rule of life John Rockefeller, the oil baron stuck to all his life, despite his billions: he remained healthy and slim and died at 93, a Methuselah's age in those distant days.

Does the finding that common cancers occur far less frequently in Okinawa than in the West (and the rest of Japan) constitute evidence that in man calorie restriction lowers the risk of cancer? The evidence is not watertight, but in man it is the best confirmation of what scientists have found in test animals: the lower the calorie–intake (and body weight) the lower the cancer incidence and conversely.

But if a low body weight protects against cancer we might all as well start sniffing cocaine. Cocaine addicts are like chain smokers, often thin as a rake.

No, the cause of the cancer protection in calorie restriction is not the low body weight (this is merely a 'symptom'), but the low glucose– and insulin levels.

This was fully explained in chapters 2 and 5.

Incidentally, the BMI of Okinawans is on the average 20.4, so well within the 'normal zone' (18.5 - 24.5).

So, is a value of 20.4 sufficient for cancer protection?

No, not for Western man who follows a different diet, as a result of which at this BMI value his glucose and insulin levels are higher than in the Okinawans. Thus it is important – as explained in chapter 6 – in addition to maintaining a low BMI and low-calorie diet to further lower the insulin level by taking a CR-mimetic (a drug that imitates the action of calorie restriction).

Currently the most effective and safe mimetic is de drug metformin, derived from the French lily, that has been used in folk's medicine since the Middle Ages.

In chapter 6 you can read everything you need to know about this preparation as protection against cancer and how to obtain it from your doctor.

I take it daily myself, not because I have diabetes, but as a powerful protection against cancer and to slow down the aging process (see chapter 5).

Why does it make sense to protect yourself against cancer when this protection is simply a matter of 'lower risk'?

An analogy may be helpful. Suppose you are a volunteer in the Korean war of 1950. You have a choice to join one of two battalions: one has a mortality rate of 50 per cent, the other of 5 per cent. Which one would you choose? If you're not suicidal probably the 5 per cent battalion, I guess. Lower risk of a bad outcome, but no guarantee!

If you can't obtain metformin there is a second choice, the nutrient supplement resveratrol, which – like metformin - is a CR-mimetic (see chapter **12**).

Chapter 8

Your body weight and cancer risk

As we have seen in chapters 3 and 6 overweight is a fertile breeding ground for cancer, a finding that prompted the oncologist professor Michael Pollak of the University of Montreal to declare: "Cancer loves the metabolic environment of the obese person."

Make sure that you maintain a 'normal' body weight, i.e. a BMI below 25.

As mentioned in chapter 7 you can have your BMI determined through 'Google', but for the sake of completeness I offer the simple formula: $BMI = G/L^2$, where G is weight in kg and L is height in meters.

So-to give a simple numerical example – if your weight is 100kg and you are 2 meter tall, then your BMI is 25 (100/4=25)

The safe zone is below 25, but (within limits) the lower the better.

Why does it make sense to protect yourself against cancer if it is just a matter of 'lower risk'?

An analogy may be helpful. You are a volunteer in the Korean war of the fifties. You may pick your choice from two battalions: one has en mortality rate of 50 per cent, the other of 5 per cent. Which on would you choose? Probably the 5 per cent battalion. Less risk of a bad ending, but no guarantee! So, the wise thing to do is find a doctor willing to prescribe metformin (coated tablets of 500mg, twice a day), just for halving your cancer risk.

No easy job, but the determined 'life-extender' will always succeed in the end. Consulting an orthomolecular doctor might be a good idea.

Chapter 9

Carbohydrates, insulin and Alzheimer's disease

The cause of Alzheimer's disease is unknown. More than half of the people with two copies of the Alzheimer's gene called ApoE4 will develop Alzheimer's, while about one-fourth of people with only one copy (25 per cent of the population) fall victim to this debilitating condition. People with no copies (hopefully you and I) have a ten per cent chance (still pretty high).

But as there are avoidable factors which greatly increase the risk of the disease you have the opportunity to considerably lower the chance of ever getting it. Dementia (whether it is true Alzheimer's or something else like small brain infarctions) frequently occurs in de elderly: between 80 and 85 twenty per cent of people are demented or growing demented, while between 85 and 90 this percentage is about forty.

Dementia also frequently occurs at younger ages and may strike anyone, even the smartest people. Let me offer an example. In my brother's debating society were two physics students who both became professor of theoretical physics, one in Amsterdam, the other in Leyden. Both became demented shortly after seventy.

Insulin increases the risk of Alzheimer's
In order not to make my story too complicated for the average reader I'll present the evidence that high insulin levels greatly increase the risk of Alzheimer's and other forms of dementia in a rather dogmatic fashion. The complete proof is presented in the medical appendix, which is also accessible to the layman by reading 'between the lines'.

Alzheimer's disease is an 'illness of civilization', just like heart disease, diabetes and obesity.

An example: the incidence of Alzheimer's among African Americans is twice that of the blacks in rural Africa.[14]

But more to the point: people with diabetes type-2 have twice the risk of Alzheimer's than non-diabetics. This has been shown for example in the well-known Rotterdam study involving 6000 older individuals.[15]

The study showed that diabetes doubled the risk of dementia (including Alzheimer's). Telling is the finding that patients who were treated with insulin ran four times the risk of dementia than non-diabetics! Treating diabetes type-2 with insulin further increases the already elevated insulin level. This in sharp contrast to the treatment with metformin and similar drugs that actually lower the insulin level (see chapter 5).

People with so-called pre-diabetes, a condition whereby the insulin level is elevated (hyperinsulinaemia) in the absence of diabetes, also run a higher risk of dementia.

On the basis of these findings it is firmly established that the higher the insulin level the greater the risk of dementia and of course the reverse: the lower the insulin level the lower the risk. As is fully discussed in chapters 2 and 5 you can achieve a low insulin level by carbohydrate restriction, possibly supported by metformin.

How does insulin act?
Feel free to skip this section since you're already motivated to restrict your carbohydrate consumption anyway in order to live longer and prevent the development of cancer (chapters 5 and 2).

As is well-know, Alzheimer's is characterized by the accumulation of so-called amyloid plaques (junk of undigested amyloid proteins) in the brain.

---

14 Hendrie, H.C. et al, "Incidence of Dementia and Alzheimer's disease in 2 Communities: Yorubu Residing in Ibadan, Nigeria, and African Americans in Indianapolis, Indiana", JAMA, 285, 739, 2001.
15 Ott, A.R.P., Diabetes Mellitus and the risk of dementia: The Rotterdam Study", Neurology, 53, 1937, 1999

The centrepiece here is a certain enzyme that is also present in the brain, the insulin degrading enzyme (IDE).

IDE is present in brain cells, the neurons, where it does two things: it breaks down insulin and it breaks down the amyloid-protein. But if the (local) insulin concentration becomes too high (like in diabetes) IDE is unable to degrade amyloid sufficiently, since the breaking down of insulin takes priority. So amyloid remains as trash in the brain cell, disrupting its function with memory loss and Alzheimer's as a sequel.

This is such a strange story that even a science fiction writer could not have invented it. But you can convince yourself by typing in Wikipedia "IDE-Alzheimer's disease": then you get all the information you will ever need! Mice, in which the IDE gene has been genetically removed, exhibit 50 per cent less amyloid degradation, resulting in amyloid accumulation and dementia (which can also be established in animals).

Besides insulin, other factors such as glycation (AGEs) are involved in Alzheimer's, but this is a matter for the medical appendix.

Medical Appendix

A practical problem with dementia is that the underlying cause is often hard to establish.
A well-known complication in diabetes is the so-called vascular dementia which can easily be confused with Alzheimer's. Vascular dementia results from a disruption of the blood flow to the brain, with or without a number of strokes, big or small (CVA, or, cerebral vascular attacks). In most cases, both with or without diabetes, a mixed picture is present: vascular dementia and Alzheimer's inextricably mixed.

Amyloid accumulation is like atherosclerosis a 'normal' process during aging. It is absent under 50, while after that age the incidence (frequency of occurrence) gradually rises, until it reaches about 40 per cent between 80-90. Only above a certain threshold level amyloid accumulation leads to Alzheimer's.

As you know Alzheimer's is pathologically characterized by two phenomena: 1) neurofibrillary tangles' (sticking together of protein threads) in the neurons an 2) amyloid plaque outside the neurons.
The current view is that these amyloid plaques (the real culprits) are formed by the combined action of glycation (see chapter 6) and insulin, 'coincidentally' the two characteristics of diabetes type-2 and related conditions such as pre-diabetes, hyperinsulinaemia and the metabolic syndrome.
Let us begin with glycation and its end product, AGEs (Advanced Glycation End products), which are fully discussed in chapter 6.

As is well-known and almost self-evident, accumulation of AGEs in all organs and tissues is present in diabetes.

But AGEs are also found in amyloid plaques, even in 'immature' plaques, indicating that they are causally involved in the early stages. Because AGEs also promote crosslinking (the sticking together of protein threads to form a tangle) amyloid is hard to remove, while enzymes, among which IDE, involved in the removal of amyloid, are inactivated. To make matters worse glycation leads to the production of free radicals (very aggressive) that further damage the neurons. The significance of IDE has been explained earlier in this chapter. Here I'll mention only a definitive study of the leading researcher in this field, Dr. Suzanne Graft. When insulin was intravenously given to elderly people the amyloid concentration in their liquor cerebralis increased proportional to the insulin concentration. The reason is that IDE is overtaxed by its primary task to break down local insulin; so, less is available to remove amyloid.

It may be mentioned in passing that Dr. Graft also showed that insulin in the short run actually improves memory and cognitive functions. Chronic long lasting hyperinsulinaemia is however the main cause of the manifestation of this disease.

In a 2004 paper the Harvard neurologists Dennis Selkoe and Rudolph Tanzi wrote that "drugs that can increase IDE-activity decrease the amyloid level in the human brain."

This implies that any measure that decreases the insulin level in the long run is effective since more IDE becomes available for the removal of amyloid.

This 'preventive therapy' already exists and is at your disposal: less carbohydrate.

Chapter 10

About baking, broiling, cheese and breakfast cereals: careful!

I have lots of friends - 800 just on Facebook alone - but I'm afraid that I - on the principle of 'Kill the messenger' - will have few friends left after the bad news in this chapter.

In chapter 6 I discussed the concept 'glycation' and its end products AGEs (advanced glycation products). As you know this is the process of 'caramelization', whereby sugars stick to proteins, resulting in the formation of harmful AGEs (junk). Well, the same process occurs when you strongly heat proteins, as in baking and broiling. Although you don't taste it, your succulent beefsteak also contains sugars. As a result of the intense heat they will attach themselves to the proteins, thus producing the nice brown colour crust and flavour through glycation. When glycation occurs in the body as in diabetes patients it is called endogenous glycation (endo=inside). When it happens outside the body it is called exogenous glycation (exo=outside).

The way you cook determines the formation of AGEs. Cooking at high temperatures, as in baking, barbecuing, broiling, roasting, braising, magnetron increases the formation of AGEs. Cooking in water or steaming is safer as the temperature does not exceed 100° Celsius, the boiling point of water. When food becomes brown (browning) during cooking, it means that its AGEs content has increased. Since most *fast foods* and pre-packaged foods are browned this is an additional reason to avoid them.

How harmful are AGEs in our food, mostly as the result of baking and broiling?

To give you an impression: in the questionnaire about 'biological age' in the book The Immortality Edge by the prominent scientist professor Michael Fossel[16] you subtract 100 points if you suffer from coronary disease. If you eat baked or broiled food more than twice a week you must also subtract 100 points! So, obviously AGEs are very harmful. In this context it is worth mentioning that Dutch scientists have shown that the AGEs-content of blood is a very reliable predictor of the prognosis of chronic heart failure.[17]

The higher the AGEs content, the worse the prognosis.

Telling is the finding that mice who receive food containing half the AGEs content of their usual food live on the average 15 per cent longer. Translated to man this would mean that in the Netherlands our mean lifespan would increase from the current 80 years to 92 years if everyone would consume 50 per cent less AGEs.[18]

This finding alone shows the enormous contribution of AGEs to the acceleration of the aging process.

Unfortunately AGEs content is not only high in baked food, but also in cheese, sausages and breakfast cereals. An example: cheese contains more AGEs than broiled or roasted chicken breast (which contains six times more AGEs than boiled chicken breast).[19]

So, eat cheese in moderation, not because of its saturated fat content, which is unimportant (see chapter 11), but because of its AGEs content.

Incidentally, this reminds me of a patient of mine, a man in his fifties, who told me one day that he had been diagnosed with Alzheimer's. He said," It must be from all that cheese. I have always been very fond of cheese." In chapter 9 the link between AGEs and Alzheimer's is fully discussed. This anecdote proves nothing but makes you wonder in the light of our present knowledge.

---

16 The Immortality Edge '' by Michael Fossel, Greta Blackburn and David Woynarowski
17 Hartog, J.W.L., e.a. ,"Clinical and prognostic value of advanced glycaemic end products (AGEs) in chronic heart failure", European Heart Journal, 28, 2879, 2007.
18 Cai,W., e.a., Am.J.Pathol., 170, 1893, 2007.
19 Goldberg, T., e .a., J. Am. Diet Assoc., 104, 1287, 2004.

If all this is so harmful to our health how come I have never heard or read about it, you may want to know. It is indeed a new paradigm (insight) in medicine and it is all about techniques to determine AGEs quantitatively. These tests - e.g. the CML test - have only become widely available in the 21st century.

What is the most dangerous place in your house? The bathroom? Breaking your neck, drowning? No, the kitchen, not because of fire hazard, but because most of us are daily mixing poison without being aware of it: AGEs.

What is the solution for the meat eater?
Boiling or steaming beefsteak? No more meat, only boiled eggs? Of course this is not an option for the 'normal' person. But forewarned, forearmed. Preparing the meat (including chicken) in the shortest possible time and at the lowest possible temperature and definitely rather medium-rare than well-done.

The 'vitalist' (life-extender) has, in the light of our present knowledge, only a limited choice: to avoid as much as possible food with a substantial AGEs content, and as to cooking: no more than twice a week baking and roasting.

Addendum
According to the American scientist, Professor M.G. Enig, one of the greatest authorities on fats (see her book 'Facts and Fats') the following fats and oils can be safely used for baking:

Corn oil, olive oil, peanut oil, butter, coconut oil, lard and palm oil.
Don't be afraid of saturated fats (saturated fatty acids). Professor Enig comments: "The assertion that saturated fat is the cause of heart disease is just dead wrong. The suggestion of harmful effects has been created by the margarine producers, who will go to any length to have their products successfully compete with butter,

lard and tallow. Eventually the idea is raised to a dogma by repeating it year after year."

The only fats you should really be afraid of are the so-called trans-fats (trans-fatty acids), the result of the artificial *hydrogenation process* used in the production of margarines. To be on the safe side it is better to use butter than margarine, although currently most margarines contain far less trans-fatty acids than before, as a result of industrial auto-regulation brought about by the efforts of the Dutch scientist professor Katan, the American scientist professor Enig and other researchers in the field.

Medical Appendix

In the appendixes of chapters 5 and 6 some aspects of the actions of glycation have already been discussed.

What follows is a brief addition with some overlap. For the sake of brevity I will present the material point by point.

1. Biomarkers for AGEs are among others CML (carboxmethyl-lysine) and methylglyoxal.

2. AGEs derived from food (exogenous glycation) exert their harmful effects via two paths: a) by deposition outside the cells and damaging protein structures, e.g. cross-linking of collagen, etc. and b) via the AGE receptor in the cell membrane, called RAGE. The interaction of AGE with the receptor RAGE (key and lock) results via a number of intermediate steps, in the production of well-known inflammation factors such as cytokines and growth factors. The result is chronic inflammation (a main player in aging) and oxidative stress. In this context it is relevant to mention that researchers of the National Institute of Aging and the Mount Sinai School of Medicine have shown in 2010 that an AGES-restricted diet (containing 50 per cent less AGEs than the normal AGEs-rich diet by cooking at low temperature), after three months resulted in a spectacular improvement of the biomarkers of inflammation, as compared to the control group. As you know inflammation (the non-infectious type) is a major cause of (accelerated) aging.

3. AGEs results in the stiffening of arteries, atherosclerosis (plaque-formation) and the loss of endothelial function. A large number of age-related diseases, including, Alzheimer's,

Parkinson's disease (chapter 9), rheumatoid arthritis, kidney failure, cataract, etc. are caused or aggravated by AGEs (glycation).

4. Approximately 10 to 30 per cent of exogenous AGEs are resorbed by the body. One third of this is excreted by the kidneys. The rest remains in the body.

5. The greatest AGEs polluters in the Western diet are milk and milk products (CML), meat and bread (melanoidins). Excessive ingestion of fruit is to be avoided, since fructose possesses a far stronger glycation action than glucose. Obviously, pastries, cake, pizza, etc. are, due to the method of preparation, rich sources of AGEs.

6. It is no exaggeration to say that the glycation problem (both exogenous and endogenous) represents the greatest medical challenge of the 21st century.

7. The radical solution? Little milk and milk products, less bread, stewing your meat and not too much sweet fruit. Whether the reader will heed this advice is another matter ...

Chapter 11

Cholesterol, saturated fats, statins and your heart

Year after year we are being frightened by the medical authorities about 'cholesterol', the alleged El Capone among the nutrients and blood test results. There is no smoke without fire. A very high cholesterol value, like in the inborn condition *familiar hypercholesterolaemia,* can be dangerous and increase the risk of a heart attack or stroke. For ordinary people like you and I both cholesterol in food and in the blood is of little importance, as statistical studies demonstrate. The cholesterol hype has little to do with science, but everything with medical politics, brain-washing of doctors and the public and billions in the sale of pills (Lipitor) and 'healthy' margarines.

How does Defares dare to allege such nonsense, entirely at odds with the advice of my cardiologist and family doctor?

Clearly, I must give this thesis a solid scientific underpinning.

Let me start with a similar medical fallacy that has been promoted as the gospel truth for more than a century. Until recently it was 'a well-established fact' that stomach ulcer was caused by stress and hyperactivity of the so-called vagus nerve. Big Pharma earned billions from symptom-suppressing drugs that neutralised the vagus activity.

But the theory was wrong: the cause was a bacterium, Helicobacter pylori. The Australian doctor Barry Marshall, who presented his 'absurd' theory in 1983 was booed off the stage, totally ignored. He writes in his autobiography: "My results were challenged and not believed, not on the basis of science, but because they simply couldn't be true."

In 1984 he used himself as guinea pig: he swallowed a colony of the Helicobacter Bacilla, promptly became very ill and the biopsy showed the ulcer and the bacterial invasion. Later he could demonstrate in a double-blind study that antibiotics treatment permanently cured the condition. The newspaper headings screamed, "Guinea pig doctor discovers new cause of stomach ulcer and its cure."

In 2005 he received the Nobel Prize for his epoch-making discovery.

A patient of mine, ex- top manager at Pfizer, told me that Pfizer had just invested a billion dollars in developing a new 'anti-vagus pill' when the bacterial cause of stomach ulcer was very reluctantly accepted by the medical authorities and the industry. A full-blown disaster for Big Pharma at the time!

The lesson: 1) you can earn billions on the basis of a wrong theory and 2) the wrong theory may be granted a very long life.

The big difference between this example and the cholesterol hypothesis is however that in the case of the stomach ulcer the pharm-industry could flourish by treating the symptoms, while with the cholesterol hypothesis no symptoms need to be treated, but only people's fears need to be manipulated. An easier way to make lots of money is not conceivable!

The hypothesis that 'too much 'cholesterol is the cause of atherosclerosis and a risk factor for cardio-vascular diseases is such a false theory. As we will see the cause of atherosclerosis is (non-infectious) low-level inflammation, while cholesterol is unimportant as a risk factor in cardiovascular narrowing and heart attacks.

Origin of the 'cholesterol hypothesis'
In the field of medicine the United States always takes the lead. What is there regarded as medical truth gets into the textbooks and is accepted as gospel truth worldwide.

The cholesterol theory began with Dr. Ancel Keys' prospective Seven Countries Study in which populations of seven countries (Italy, Yugoslavia, Greece, Finland, The Netherlands, Japan and the USA) were studied with regard to eating habits (saturated fat), cholesterol levels and cardiac mortality. The results were impressive. Expressed in deaths per decade, there were 9 cardiac deaths per ten thousand in Crete, as compared to 992 for the lumberjacks and farmers in Finland. In between were the Japanese with 66 per ten thousand, Italian railway workers with 290 and American railway workers with 570.

According to Keys the Seven Countries Study taught us three things: 1) cholesterol levels predicted cardiac risk, 2) the amount of saturated fat in our food predicted cholesterol levels and heart ailments and 3) mono-unsaturated fat (olive oil) protects against heart trouble. This would be the reason according to Keys that both Finnish lumberjacks as well as Crete farmers could eat a diet containing 40 per cent fat, but could show such enormous differences in heart disease–incidence.

That saturated fat does not result in high blood cholesterol or cardiac mortality was already shown in chapter 4 by the fact that the Masai, a nomadic tribe in Kenia and northern Tanzania, exclusively live on milk, meat, blood and animal fat. Their cholesterol level is normal and cardio-vascular disease is totally absent among the Masai. Dr. George Mann who studied the Masai extensively in the seventies reports that they have the highest intake of saturated fat and cholesterol "ever recorded".

As Gary Taubes, science editor, e.g. of the leading science journal *Science,* says: "Despite the legendary status of the Seven Countries Study it was fatally flawed." Taubes observes: "To begin with, Keys chose seven countries that he knew would support this hypothesis. Had Keys chosen at random, or, for example, France and Switzerland, instead of Finland and Japan, then he would not have found any effect of saturated fat and the so-called *French Paradox* – a country that consumes a lot of saturated fat but with relatively little heart disease – would not have existed.[20]

Incidentally, recent data of the WHO's MONICA-study, that studies the prevalence of cardiovascular disease and its risk factors worldwide, show that the country with the lowest mean cholesterol value (5.3), Russia, has the highest mortality from coronary heart disease (800), while the country with the highest mean cholesterol level (6.5), Switzerland, has the lowest heart-related mor-

---

20   Taubes, Gary, Good Calories, Bad Calories, Alfred A. Knopf, 2007, p. 32.

tality (160). This recent finding is obviously completely at odds with Keys' hypothesis and disproves it.

Despite the fact that 'hard' scientists (statisticians, etc.) attach little significance to epidemiological studies where the differences are small (as when someone who eats a lot of fat has twice the risk of getting a heart condition; this in contrast to smokers, who have a 30 times higher risk of lung cancer), the Seven Countries Study constitutes the foundation of the 'cholesterol hypothesis 'of the medical community. The edifice rests on quicksand, as we will see.

The Medical-Industrial Complex

In his farewell speech president Eisenhower warned of the dangers of the military-industrial complex, the incestuous relationship between the military elite and the arms industry. The same close relationship exists between the medical elite and the pharmaceutical and food industry. As an outsider you don't have the faintest idea how close the links are between clinicians and academic researchers on the one hand and the industry on the other. With regard to a subject like antibiotics this is not very serious: at most antibiotics are too often prescribed. With regard to cholesterol and related subjects (statins, like Lipitor) the situation is very different. Big Pharma and Big Food smell billions: science is completely subordinated to propaganda, sales promotion and profit seeking and not only the public, but doctors as well are brainwashed by an industry adept at throwing dust in doctors' eyes, leaving aside the financial links between professors and Big Pharma. (Incidentally, I was one of these professors as a younger man and was richly rewarded by Big Pharma, until I wrote an article warning against the dangers of the Pill).

Since I'm talking about myself in my days as medical researcher, many decennia ago, academic scientists could study the merits of a drug with a considerable degree of independence. Those days are long gone.

Dr. Marcia, ex editor-in-chief of the prestigious medical journal *New England Journal of Medicin* , observes:

In the past drug companies just gave money to academic medical centres to enable clinical investigators to do a study and that was it. There was a great distance. The researcher performed his experiment and published his or her results, whatever those results were. Today it is very different. Increasingly the pharmaceutical companies design the studies themselves. They own the data. Not even the researchers are given full access to the data.

The companies analyse the data and they determine whether the data are published or not. They force researchers and academic centres to sign contracts, in which they promise not to publish their work, unless explicit permission is granted by the pharmaceutical company. The pharmaceutical company determines what the data show, what conclusions are drawn and whether the data are published or not.

The medical profession has been degraded to the role of servant of Big Pharma. **Incredible, but this is the reality.** An example: virtually all medical professors of Harvard (where I have worked as a visiting lecturer) have close links with the pharmaceutical industry: they are the opinion makers.

Is there a better way to make billions from 'cholesterol' than pulling the wool over everyone's eyes, both patient's and doctor's? You don't have to cure anything, not even alleviate symptoms, just predict disaster, unless ...

Science as servant of the pharmaceutical propaganda machine. True? Of course this is an exaggeration, but for 90 per cent a reality.

But there is another obstacle for 'the truth', the wrong view of the medical authorities. After the publication of Keys study in 1970 the "Keys' diet" and the Keys' hypothesis became government policy and the darling of the American Medical Association and the American Heart Association. Loss of face from new (unwelcome) facts is sufficient reason for the authorities to adapt the facts to dogma, instead of the hypothesis to the data. All very human and understandable, but at the expense of your health and wellbeing.

So, now you're somewhat prepared to digest the following facts.

Loss of face is also the reason that the most rigorous epidemiological study ever conducted, the Framingham Heart Study, established under the auspices of the American Heart Association was never published, because the NIH (National Institutes of Health) which funded the study withheld the publication. There did appear a report in the 24th part of the bulky Framingham Report series that no one would ever read.

I'll just mention some of the findings that ran counter to the 'conventional wisdom'.

Males with a very high cholesterol level (above 300) were compared with males with very low cholesterol (less than 170). To the disappointment of the researchers there was no difference in the amount or type of fat that the two groups consumed.

A second unexpected result was that after an observation span of thirty years there was no correlation between lifespan and cholesterol in men and women over fifty.

In other words, high cholesterol has no influence on life expectancy whatsoever.

A third result was that cholesterol intake (much or little) has no influence on the cholesterol level whatsoever.

A fourth result was that there was no correlation between diet (fat, cholesterol) and heart disease.

But the Framingham study is merely the *primus inter pares* of a number of epidemiological studies (screening of the population) in 11 countries. In 2001 the so-called Cochrane Collaboration, which was established in 1991 by 27 top scientists, published an analysis of 27 publications (involving more than ten thousands subjects) that were selected from the medical literature on the basis of rigorous criteria (www.cochrane.org). The conclusion: **the diets (low in fat and/or low in cholesterol) had no effect on life expectancy and even (quote) "no significant effect on cardiac calamities."**

> The Cochrane Collaboration is an international network of more than 28,000 scientists and policy makers in 100 countries. Its main purpose is to offer objective information to doctors in order to enable them to make well-informed decisions about health-care on the basis of 'randomized controlled trials'. In 2001 the Collaboration was allotted a seat in the World Health Assembly of the World Health Organization.

I could captivate or bore you for hours with evidence of the complete incorrectness of the cholesterol hypothesis, the greatest medical deception of all times.

I'll refrain from that. I shall only mention a telling commentary from the press. In 1970 the publication of MRFIT (Multiple Risk Factor Intervention Trial) appeared, set up by the American National Heart, Lung and Blood Institute, in which 12,000 "high-risk" men were selected from among 360,000 participants. These were randomly subdivided in two groups. One group was allowed to continue to eat their usual ('normal') diet, the other was put on a stringent low-fat, low-cholesterol diet for years. End-result: there were slightly more deaths in the group on the stringent diet. In 1982 an editorial article appeared in the Wall Street Journal about this study with the heading: "Heart attacks: A Test Collapses". The Wall Street Journal is not exactly a criticaster of Big Pharma and the establishment. *Need I say more?*

Let us pause ... How then is it possible you may ask in bewilderment that doctors and medical brochures offer such 'precise' instructions to fight cholesterol?

It is like a mantra, just parrotry. I did the same before I studied the evidence. Just as the silly mantra of cardiologists: "At most three eggs a week". Absolute hogwash as attested by hundreds of studies, including the Framingham trials (see above).

But once a mantra is established in clinical medicine it is virtually impossible to get rid of it, partly due to the fact that doctors are too busy to keep up with the scientific medical literature. But of course it is all a bit more complicated than that, as we will examine ...

Of course there must be some relationship between 'cholesterol' and the risk of heart attacks etc., otherwise the cholesterol hype would never have stood the test of time. However, the connection is weak and is of consequence for 'public health' only, not for the individual.

This strategy in relation to the cholesterol theme was presented for the first time in 1981 by the British epidemiologist Geoffrey Rose and is similar to e.g. diphtheria vaccination. Before vaccination diphtheria struck 1 in 600 children in England, in other words, 599 children had to be vaccinated to save 1 child. This is called preventive medicine and is aimed at improving the health statistics of the population.

Vaccination is one thing, but to avoid eating saturated fat (cheese) for the rest of your life and swallowing a pill (statin) daily (with many side effects, some of them serious), is a different story altogether. If you're very socially minded in this regard, please do participate, but definitely not to save your own skin.

Below I'll present some reasons 'why not':

1. According to the calculations of Professor Rose (see above) only 1 male out of 50 would avoid a heart attack by avoiding eating saturated fat all his life. He states: "49 men would have to eat very differently and probably would derive no benefit from it at all."
2. If males with a heart condition (high-risk group) would swallow a statin (anti-cholesterol pill) daily for thirty years, this would lead to an average lifespan extension of two months.
3. If you're a male with established cardiovascular disease, statins lower your risk of dying with 0.66 per cent at the most (Malcolm Kendrick).
4. **If you're a man or a woman without cardiovascular disease statins extend your life with not a single day**

Worse, your life expectancy is a bit shorter. Dr. Graham Jackson concludes in the *British Journal of Pharmacology*:

When all large controlled studies are combined (this is called meta-analysis, J.G.D.), it leads to the conclusion that long-term use of statins for primary prevention of cardiovascular diseases (so, in healthy people, J.G.D.) results in a one per cent higher risk of dying within ten years relative to the placebo group.

These solid figures thus show that if you're not a heart patient there is absolutely no point in going on a 'fat-free' diet or use a statin (Lipitor, etc.) as your family doctor may insist. Knowledge is power, especially where it concerns your own body.

The question keeps nagging: "Yes, but, how about all those hard statistics? Is that not sufficient proof? They can't just have made it all up, can they?"

As a former professor in mathematical biology at the medical faculty of the University of Leyden (Holland) I can tell you on the basis of professional experience that there are two forms of lies: common lies and statistical lies. With statistics you can tell the 'ignorant public' (including patients and doctors, who are statistically illiterate) anything, and even scare them to death.

I yield the floor to Dr. Malcolm Kendrick, who illuminates this problem with a hilariously funny analogy.

Time to unveil a nice statistical game that researchers in the field of cardiovascular disease love to play. It is called: 'Data inflation-the Revenge'.

To illustrate how you can transform innocent statistics into weapons of mass destruction, I'll put the following simple question to you. What are the odds of winning the first prize in a lottery? About 1 in 15 million a week [in England, J.G.D.]. *If I would be able to increase the odds from 1 in 15 million to 1.5 in 15 million I could claim that I have increased your chance by fifty per cent. That fifty per cent represents however the relative increase of your chance. The absolute increase is 0.5 in 15,000,000, or, 1 in 30,000,000. Expressed in percentage: 0,000003.*

Suppose I tried to sell my lottery odds-increasing service to you. Which number I would probably use to bring you round? I can visualize the ad. "Would you like to be a millionaire? Yes? The world famous lottery expert Dr. Kendrick can increase your chances of winning the jackpot by fifty per cent. Oh sure, by fifty per cent! You could be the winner! The only thing you have to do is send twenty euro in a stamped envelope and you'll get advice! This is not a phoney trick, this advice works, you can count on that."

By contrast I would not be so foolish to offer my services as follows: "The desperate, lonely and hard-up Dr. Kendrick can increase your miserably small chance of winning the lottery by a meagre, hardly measurable 0.000003 per cent."

You must admit that fifty per cent sounds more impressive than 0.000003 per cent. However both figures are correct. O, yes, statistical truth, slippery as an eel!

The good and the bad cholesterol
We all know that cholesterol comes in different 'flavours': there is total cholesterol, HDL-cholesterol (the 'good') and LDL-cholesterol (the 'bad') and there is also (most people haven't heard of this) the triglycerides (blood fats, or rather fatty acids). I shall not tire you by explaining what this is all about. It is sufficient to know that total cholesterol – as the Framingham studies and scores of other epidemiological studies have shown – represents no risk factor for heart disease. So, what remains? A 'too high' LDL, a 'too low' HDL and a 'too high' triglycerides-value. What is the influence of these three factors? The National Institutes of Health (USA) financed and organised five simultaneous studies in Framingham, Puerto Rico, Honolulu, Albany and San Francisco in order to obtain an empirical answer to this burning question. The results were published in 1977. Here are the conclusions from Dr. Gordon and his team:

1. Total cholesterol is no risk factor at all for coronary heart disease.

2. LDL-cholesterol is a "marginal" risk factor.

3. Triglycerides [high values, J.G.D.] predicted coronary heart disease both in men and in women.

4. The most important risk factor was, however, the HDL-cholesterol (the good one). The higher HDL-cholesterol the lower triglycerides and the risk of heart disease. This inverse relationship between HDL and heart disease was present at all ages above 40, both in men as well as in women. Dr. Gordon reports:" Of all measured lipoproteins and lipids HDL had the greatest influence on risk."

HDL-cholesterol is the only reliable predictor of risk.
The conclusion of this study that cost 300 million dollars and has never been equalled since, is that only HDL (HDL-cholesterol) is important as a risk factor. In fact one does not need to measure triglycerides, since we know that when HDL is high, triglycerides are low and conversely.

So, of the three tests your family doctor orders, total cholesterol, LDL and HDL, only the latter is of clinical importance. Total cholesterol is completely unimportant, LDL is marginally important and HDL is important.

But here is the big problem for the pharmaceutical industry: they can make drugs that lower LDL, but (thus far) they are unable to produce drugs that significantly increase HDL.

But not to worry! The marginal influence on LDL is greatly blown up by clever statistics and *voilà*: Zocor or Lipitor for everyone!

A recent statin that strongly increases HDL has been taken off the market because of unacceptable toxicity.

Statins mainly lower LDL.

The slight increase in HDL (3-12 per cent, dependent on which brand) is a kind of side-effect. The most effective way to increase (a low) HDL is however the vitamin B, niacin, (3 grams daily), while physical exercise, diet (carbohydrates restriction), fish oil capsules and even alcohol (2 units/day) increase HDL.

There is not the slightest reason to use a statin to improve a low HDL.

Conclusion:
Statistical studies have shown that total cholesterol is meaningless, and that LDL-cholesterol is a weak predictor of heart trouble. The only serious predictor (risk–factor) is HDL: a low HDL is unfavourable. This quantity is not appreciably affected by the use of statins with their many side effects. Dietary changes and other non-pharmaceutical measures are almost always sufficient to normalize a low HDL.

Better not use statins
As you probably will not be highly motivated to use statins after having read the preceding text I'll keep the discussion of statins to a minimum. One thing is certain: they are harmful and even potentially life-threatening. It is well–established on the basis of numerous studies that the lower the cholesterol the higher the cancer risk and conversely. Very low cholesterol values (as in people who react strongly to a statin) are associated with a greatly elevated risk of cancer. One positive effect of statins has recently been found which is totally unrelated to cholesterol, but which is due to their anti-inflammatory action is that they do decrease the risk of dying from coronary heart disease. (So, this effect is independent of the cholesterol level during treatment) Wow, isn't this reason enough to use them?

No, since total mortality (all causes) remains unchanged. So, as a result of the use of statins the decrease of heart-related mortality is 'compensated' (nullified) by an increase in some other fatal condition, or conditions.

Yes, indeed, and the most frequently occurring 'extra' disease is cancer, a disease which, as noted above, increases when cholesterol decreases. The mode of action is partially known. Statins inhibit through their point of action in the liver (mevalonaat) the production of selenoproteins that offer a crucial protection against cancer, since selenium, which has a strong anti-cancer action, can only perform optimally when sufficient selenoproteins are present.

If you have a choice, dear reader, it is better to die from a heart attack then from cancer!

But there is no need to make such a hard choice as there are much saver ways to protect yourself against cardio-vascular disease than statins, such as omega-3, a low-carb diet, etc.

Lipitor and other statins
The following passage is taken from Dr. M. Kendrick's book *The Cholesterol Hype*.

The greatest drawback of statins is not that they kill a few hundred people every year worldwide, the problem is that they cause a gigantic burden of treacherous side-effects that for the most part go unrecognized, or are persistently denied by doctors. Are you tired? Well, you're getting on in age, aren't you. Muscle aches, joint pains? Cheer up, Mrs Johnson, we're all afflicted by it at times. Even if you list the catalogue of well-documented side-effects most doctors refuse to believe that they are in any way connected to the statin you're taking. (end quote)

Let me offer a personal observation. Mrs L., who has been taking care of the manuscripts of my books for donkey's years, had been on statins for some time. Before my very eyes she changed from an energetic, alert seventy-year-old woman into a rambling, unsteady wreck, who, when I called her on phone, stumbled out of her chair to pick up the phone with great difficulty, leaving me annoyed after a long wait. She had a catalogue of vague complaints and actually felt rotten, both physically and mentally. At the time I had no idea she was on Lipitor. Bemused, I asked her. Yes, she had been taking it now for some months. I advised her to stop. Within 2 weeks she was her ebullient old self again, a true 'resurrection'.

Statins are potentially very harmful, even if it were just for the fact that they suppress the body's own production of the life-giving co-enzyme Q10 in the liver. This could actually lead to heart failure in the elderly because Q10 is essential for the production of energy in the mitochondria, the energy batteries of our cells, including the heart cells.

For a complete discussion of all the misery you may expect from the use of statins I would like to refer the reader to the ultimate book on the subject, *STATIN DRUGS Side Effects* by Dr. Duane Graveline, astronaut, physician, scientist, who had experienced these 'side effects' himself, leaving him a zombie. For anyone who considers taking statins this book is required reading. It will make your hair stand on end ...

Chapter 12

Resveratrol: life-extender and CR-mimetic?

In chapter 5 the concept of CR-mimetic has been discussed at length. To refresh your memory: calorie restriction or CR, whereby the test animal is given 30 per cent less calories than it would normally consume, is the ideal method to strongly inhibit the aging process and extend life span by 20 - 50 per cent, depending on the species used.

But since no one can stick to such a diet scientists have searched for substances that copy the biological mode of action of CR (mimic), hence the term 'mimetic'. This would enable people to obtain the same results as CR just by taking a daily pill, so, without getting hungry.

As we have seen metformin is an excellent CR-mimetic. But all ways lead to Rome and one of them is the well-known substance found in red wine, resveratrol. But you would need to drink hundreds of bottles of wine to get your daily supply. So, it must be taken as a supplement.

Apart from being a strong anti-oxidant resveratrol is also a CR-mimetic. So, it imitates the anti-aging actions of drastic calorie restriction. Just like other CR-mimetics (e.g. metformin) resveratrol acts by lowering the insulin and glucose levels, but the point of action is not – as in the case of metformin - TOR, but SIRT1.[21]

After this very obscure remark I'll limit myself here to three points:

---

21 SIRT or sirtuin, is the abbreviated term of 'silent information regulator proteins'. SIRT1 plays a role in aging, while its equivalent, SIRT2, when activated, doubles life-span in lower life-forms such as yeast and certain mini-worms (C.elegans). Resveratrol enhances the activity of SIRT1 in mammals, including man.

1. How is the uptake and biological availability of resveratrol?
2. What is the correct dosage?
3. Which brands are sufficiently effective?

ad 1) **The biological activity**

Although resveratrol is well-absorbed by the gut, the resveratrol level in the blood is very low. How can this be? The reason is that resveratrol mainly accumulates in the cells that line the intestines. The contrast between the effectiveness shown in animal experiments and the low blood values of resveratrol can be explained from the fact that its break-down products (so-called metabolites) are also biologically effective and can e.g. reduce chronic inflammation.[22]

An important practical point is that the well -known supplement quercitin strengthens the biological activity of resveratrol.[23]

So it is a good idea to take resveratrol in combination with quercitin (which protects against cancer), as I do.

Besides its activating action on SIRT1 (see footnote 23) resveratrol also activates the enzyme AMPK, the key enzyme that is activated by calorie-restriction and the target of metformin (see chapter 5). Moreover, AMPK and SIRT1 reinforce each other's CR-mimetic actions according to a 2009 study of Sirtris scientists (Sirtris was founded by Professor David Sinclair of Harvard).

ad 2) **The optimal dosage**

Joseph Maroon mentions in his book about resveratrol 'The Longevity Factor' that in June 2006 fifteen scientists led by Dr. Sinclair Weinbruch reported their results with very low doses of resveratrol. They used a dosage of 4-9 mg/kg

---

[22] According to David Sinclair (Harvard) and others the metabolites of resveratrol activate the SIRT1 enzyme and thus reduce inflammation.
[23] This is due to the suppression of the attachment of the sulfa molecule to cholesterol in the liver.

bodyweight in mice and found that this low dose partially imitates (mimics) calorie-restriction and delays aging.

According to their calculation the corresponding dosage for man is only of the order of 50 mg (very low and very affordable).

The researchers conclude in their paper, *"Resveratrol in dosages that can easily be attained in humans meets the definition of a supplement or food that mimics a number of aspects of calorie restriction."*

This is good news. Most resveratrol researchers (including Professor David Sinclair of Harvard) however take higher doses: 200-1000 mg/day.

It may be mentioned in passing that resveratrol, even when taken in much higher doses (up to 5000 mg/day), has no appreciable side effects.

ad 3) Since resveratrol is highly susceptible to oxidation and most resveratrol brands do not activate the crucial SIRT1 enzyme according to tests carried out in the Anti-aging Laboratory in Harvard, the warning "Caveat Emptor" (buyer beware) should be sounded.

Activation of SIRT1 is a pre-condition for the anti-aging action of resveratrol).

On the basis of this and other considerations the choice of the hundreds of different resveratrol preparations on the market is a maze. As a short guideline I recommend four excellent products (google):

Longivinex
Biotivia
RevGenetics
Life Extension Foundation

Their resveratrol preparation meets the two minimum requirements: production in an oxygen-free environment and certified activation of sirtuin (SIRT1).

Biotivia offers the best buy. Longivinex has the best scientific background (Its product *Advantage* contains quercitin, which – as mentioned - enhances its action).

Metformin or resveratrol?
The answer is: 'both'. Metformin's positive action on lifespan has been demonstrated in mammals. This has not been achieved for resveratrol, which only partially mimics the effect of calorie restriction. While the protective effect of metformin against cancer has been shown in population studies, in the case of resveratrol this has only been shown in animal experiments and – *in vitro* - in human cancer cell lines where resveratrol inhibits growth.

Medical Appendix

Resveratrol protects the heart and offers protection against atherosclerosis.

It has been known for well over seventy–five years that CR (calorie restriction), offers protection against cardiovascular disease and atherosclerosis, both in test animals and humans.

It is now well-established that this action takes place via the enzyme SIRT1. SIRT1 is the point of action of the CR-mimetic resveratrol, i.e. resveratrol enhances the action of SIRT1. That's all you need to know. The protective action of resveratrol has been shown in a large number of recent studies. It suffices to demonstrate the protective role of SIRT1. As an illustration I mention the telling titles of three research papers:

1. SIRT1 regulates aging and resistance to oxidative stress in the heart (Alcendor, R.R. e. m. *Circulation Research,* 100, 1512, 2007)
2. SIRT1 protects the heart from aging and stress (Hsu, C.P. e.m. *Biological Chemistry,* 189, 221, 2008)
3. SIRT1. A new strategy to prevent atherosclerosis (Brandes, R.P. *Cardiovascular Research,* 80, 163, 2008)

In connection with atherosclerosis it is of interest that SIRT1 regulates the production of NO in the endothelial cells lining the arteries and thus plays a very important role in inhibiting the development of atherosclerosis (see chapter 15 for a full discussion of the role of endothelial cells).

The protective role of SIRT1 (and thus of resveratrol) in atherosclerosis acts via a number of mechanisms, among which:

- suppression of inflammation in arteries

- reduction of cell senescence in smooth muscle cells

- promoting angiogenesis (the formation of new blood vessels as bypass at an occlusion

The ability of SIRT1 to inhibit inflammation, a major cause of atherosclerosis, has been shown in experiments in which isolated macrophages and endothelial cells had been treated by SIRT1 activators (including resveratrol). This resulted in much lower levels of (inflammation inducing) cytokines. The action of SIRT1 (activation) on NO production is very important. Endothelial NO synthase, an enzyme that generates NO, is both athero-protective as well as blood vessel dilating (see chapter 15).

Chapter 13

Telomeres: the 'time clock' of your life

Perhaps this chapter is (with chapter 14) the most important one of this book, if you're actively interested in 1) slowing down aging, 2) extending your lifespan and 3) rejuvenating your tissues and organs, hence, yourself.

But, as I mentioned in chapter 5, it is sometimes necessary to descend to the smallest unit of your body, your body cell. We have some 30 trillion body cells, that we cannot see without a microscope, but whose secrets our clever scientists have largely revealed.

Have a nice cup of coffee and listen to this amazing story that may drastically change your life.

But first an observation. In the foregoing chapters I have referred to such preparations as metformin and resveratrol as 'life-extenders'.

How about the so-called telomerase-activators that are discussed in this chapter and in chapter 14?

Is that 'more of the same'?

The answer is 'No'. The reason is this. Metformin and related substances mimic calorie restriction, which in test animals achieves an increase in average lifespan of 50 per cent at most. So, in man this would, theoretically speaking, mean an (average) lifespan of 120 years.

Telomerase, the miracle enzyme that the body cell can (in principle) produce, makes the cell 'immortal'. That means that a drug that is able to fully activate the production of telomerase by the cell, can make the cell immortal and thus (theoretically) make man immortal.

To be more specific: CR-mimetics can theoretically keep man '120 years young' at the maximum, while telomerase activators (the theme of chapters 13 and 14) are in principle able to keep humans in good shape until they reach the ripe age of a thousand years or more. Science fiction? No, only still way into the future, since the present generation of TA activators (TA-65, etc.) are still in the toddler stage.

In 2009 three molecular biologists, Elizabeth Blackburn, Carol Greider and Jack Szostak received the Nobel Prize for the discovery of the enzyme telomerase, which, in a heading in Time magazine was dubbed the Methuselah enzyme. Why? Because if it is fully produced in our body cells (like in the germ cells) our cells would live forever and so would we. Then we'll 'never' die or live as long as Methuselah. It is the expectation of prominent DNA scientists (molecular biologists) that a hundred years from now a lifespan of 500-1000 years can be realized. According to these scientists the current product at our disposal (TA-65) to activate telomerase and thus lengthen our telomeres may enable those who start using it at middle age to live in good health till 120-150 years. At least if the results of animal experiments in rats and other mammals are a reliable guide.

Warning: sometimes I'll say things three times. Why this repetition? Because, as the mad Bellman in Lewis Carroll's tale "The Hunting of the Snark" says: *I'll tell you thrice, what I tell you three times is true.* "

Cell division and telomeres

Our body cells are only able to divide a limited number of times, in contrast to cancer cells, bacteria and germ cells. To offer a round figure: 60 times. Why is this? In the words of the Nobel laureate Elizabeth Blackburn: "Because each cell possesses a time-clock".

This time-clock is the telomere, the cap at the ends of chromosomes (under the microscope a 'worm', consisting mainly of a piece of DNA). If you compare a chromosome to a shoelace, then the telomere is the little piece of plastic at its ends. At each cell division the telomere becomes a bit shorter and after 60 cell divisions the telomere is 'no more': gone. The result: the cell can no longer divide and either dies or stays around as a 'poisonous' old cell, called senescent cell (*senex* = old).

Yes, the telomere functions as a time-clock. After each cell division it gets a bit shorter and after sixty cell divisions it is all over. Metaphorically: 60 seconds have elapsed; the process comes to a halt!

Perhaps the following picture is helpful. Consider the telomere to be a string with 60 beads. At each cell division a bead falls off. So, after 60 cell divisions all sixty beads have fallen off the string. End of the story.

But suppose the telomere has initially 120 beads instead of 60. Then the cell would be able to divide 120 times.

Another possibility to allow the cell to divide more often than 60 times is that each time a bead falls of, a 'fairy' picks it up and threads it back to the string.

In terms of the time-clock it comes down to pushing the hand back one second each time the hand moves forward one second (This picture was used by professor Blackburn in her acceptance speech in Stockholm). Thus the time-clock never reaches the end; the telomere is never 'finished': cell division continues indefinitely.

This second possibility, putting back a fallen bead, is the theme of our story. Who, no what, is the 'fairy' who puts back the bead or may even thread back several fallen beads?

The answer is short and sweet: it is the enzyme telomerase that every body cell can *potentially* produce.

Why doesn't it happen? Because – to use a metaphor - the telomere tap in all your 200 different types of body cells is shut off.

Let me refresh your memory. As you know every cell in your body has the same DNA, a string of some 20,000 genes that constitutes the blueprint of life. The telomerase gene (when it is 'open') gives the instruction to the cell to produce the enzyme telomerase. Then the cell becomes immortal: it continues to divide indefinitely given the right conditions. Fantasy? No, reality. We have some 200 different types of body cells: liver cells, brain cells, muscle cells, etc.

But we also have a very special kind of cells, the sex cells. In the male they produce the spermatocytes. Our sex cells are immortal.

When you grow muscle cells on a Petrie dish in the lab they can only divide 60 times. Then they (usually) die.

When you grow sex cells, they continue to divide indefinitely, just like cancer cells: they are immortal.

What do cancer cells and sex cells have in common? You guessed it: they produce the Methuselah enzyme telomerase in abundance because their telomerase gene is fully 'open' (active). It is that simple.

Does the fact that a cancer cell produces plenty of telomerase mean that telomerase is dangerous? By no means, for then the sex cell would also be dangerous, which is not the case at all. To set your mind fully at rest: embryonic stem cells continue to divide indefinitely in the laboratory because they produce plenty of telomerase. Only when this cell in the embryo receives a signal to specialize the telomerase tap (gene) is cut off and it becomes mortal. To repeat: all cells have the same DNA, so the same genes. So our 200 different cell types all possess the telomerase gene. This gene is in the 'sleeping mode' ('tap closed'). It is the challenge of science and bio-technology to open this tap (activate the gene), so our body cells also become immortal, or, at the least, double their number of divisions from 60 to 120, enabling us to become 250 years young.

Note. In the frame below it is explained by analogy why telomeres *have to* get shorter at each cell division.

About telomere shortening

When a cell divides, the genetic material of the cell (DNA) has to be copied. This process is called DNA replication. This replication is carried out by certain enzymes. Since these enzymes are unable to copy a DNA string all the way to the end a bit of DNA is lost during replication.

Fortunately this is not a piece of DNA containing genes, for then genetic material would be lost at each cell division.

No, what is lost is 'non-genetic' material, a piece of the telomere, the piece of plastic at the end of the shoe lace, the 'cap' at both ends of the chromosome, which is a piece of DNA.

To give you an idea why this piece *must* be lost I present an analogy.

As an analogy you could think of DNA as a long row of bricks and the DNA replication as a bricklayer, who, walking backwards, puts a new layer on top of the bricks (of the first layer). So he cannot copy the last brick without him falling off. So the second layer is one brick shorter than the first. This is repeated: the third layer is again one brick shorter than the second row, etc. And at a certain moment only one brick remains. The process comes to an end. The bricklayer is no longer able to put a brick in place; the cell can no longer copy the DNA, because the telomere is 'too short'.

Each time our cells divide and our chromosomes replicate our telomeres get shorter. At fertilization (the start of life) the telomere has a length of 15,000 nucleotides (each cell has 46 chromosomes, so 92 telomeres). During foetal development the cells multiply furiously, so at birth out telomeres have shrunken to a length of 10,000 nucleotides.

During our lifetime they continue to shorten, since (most) cells continue to divide. When their telomeres have reached a length of 5000 nucleotides, our cells can no longer divide and we die of 'old age'. This occurs after about 60 cell divisions.

It goes without saying that the older you are the fewer cell divisions are left to occur. This has been demonstrated. When you grow cells of a forty-year-old person in the lab they can divide less often than those of a twenty-year-old, while those of a 80-year-old person much less often than those of a forty-year-old.

The remaining 'division-capacity' is independent of time. If a cell can only divide 20 times in the lab, this will be also the case when you preserve the cell in deep-freeze and 'awaken' it a century later: then it also divides no more than 20 times.

Leonard Hayflick, a scientist of near-mythical stature in this field, had shown in the middle of the last century that our cells can divide only a limited number of times (about 60 times); only the cells of the foreskin can divide 50 per cent longer, 90 times, (which again shows the superiority of me and my brothers).

The cause is the ticking time-clock, the telomere shortening.

If we can reverse it (telomere *elongatio*n) the cell can divide more often or even continue to divide without end: the Holy Grail of molecular biology. For then each time the hand of the time-clock moves forward it is pushed back.

As has been mentioned in the frame, the telomere consists of (chemical) units, represented by the letter sequence TTAGGG.

If chemistry is not your strongest subject you can think of a telomere as a very long string of beads of three different colours, terracotta (T), amber (A), and green (G): so, TTAGGG, TTAGGG, TTAGGG …

If we call this letter combination a 'unit', then at birth your telomere had a length of about 10,000 units. And now? Depending on a number of factors like your age, somewhere between 8,000 and 5,000. When your telomeres have shortened to 5,000 you're dead. Your cells can no longer divide. Then they either die or hang around as sick and noxious 'old' cells, called senescent cells (which means 'old' in Latin).

We are as old as our cells.

Telomere length therapy
As I said earlier our sex cells (also called germ cells) are 'immortal'. Under the right laboratory conditions they will continue to divide indefinitely on the Petrie dish. Their telomeres do not get shorter thanks to the presence of the enzyme telomerase in the cell.

The solution for radical life extension is to get this miracle enzyme in all our body cells and then our cells will live on for ever and so will we!

But how is this achieved?

Nature offers the solution. All cells have the same DNA, the genetic blueprint passed on by our parents. This contains some 20,000 genes and one gene is the telomerase gene. This is nothing but an instruction for the production of the enzyme telomerase (enzymes are the workers producing everything in the cell, even your hair). As stated above the telomerase gene is in virtually all body cells in a 'dormant state', there is a lid on it, so to speak, or, 'the telomerase tap is turned off'. In principle all sleeping genes can be awakened. How?

The gene is inactive if it is covered by a protein (lid)[24]

> **"Proofs of Principle"**
> The following is taken from the book **CURING AGING** from the leading scientist Dr. William Andrews. Dr. Andrews has acquired 40 patents on telomerase.
>
> There is a plan available to activate telomerase in our body cells. But how will it work out? Will it cure aging? Thus far all signs indicate that this is indeed the case: telomerase is very probably the cure for aging.
>
> In 1987 scientists implanted the telomerase gene in normal human skin cells that were grown on a Petrie dish. When they established that, as expected, the telomerase enzyme was produced by the cells, they also observed that the skin cells became immortal: there was no limit to the number of times these cells could multiply. When the length of the telomeres in these 'telomerised cells' was examined, the scientists were surprised to find that the telomeres not only stopped getting shorter; they became longer. The critical question then was: did the cells actually become younger?

---

24   In fact there are one or more locations beside the telomerase gene that serve as a binding location for the protein. When this so-called suppressor protein is attached to these locations the cell cannot produce telomerase.

A few years later scientists put the telomerase gene in human skin cells that already had very short telomeres. These cells were then grown into skin on the back of mice. As one would expect the skin from the cells that had not received the telomerase gene looked like old skin. It was wrinkled, blistered easily and had the gene-expression of old skin.

The skin derived from cells that had received the telomerase gene, however, looked young. It behaved like young skin and, what was very important, the gene expression patterns analysed by the DNA Array Chip analysis was virtually identical to the gene expression patterns of young skin. This was the first time that scientists had demonstrably reversed aging in human cells.

Would this idea be applicable to living organisms? In November 2008 scientists published an article in which it is mentioned that they had created cloned mice from mouse cells that contained the implanted telomerase gene that continuously produced telomerase. These mice turned out to live 50 per cent longer than cloned mice from cells that did not contain this telomerase gene.

It is getting increasingly evident that the prevention of telomere shortening could be the best way to increase human lifespan to beyond the (currently) theoretical maximal lifespan of 125 years.

To what extent it may increase human lifespan nobody knows, but a healthy, youthful life up to 250, 500 or even 1000 years is - from a scientific perspective - a realistic possibility. Further research is required to settle this question. (Unquote.)

The experimental evidence that telomerase activation extends life continues to accumulate, although 'immortality' has only been demonstrated in lower organisms, like flatworms. In 2012 British scientists of the university of Nottingham have shown that the flatworm increases the activity of the telomerase gene when it regenerates, resulting in the stem cells maintaining their telomere length when they divide to replace tissues.

Conclusion: because flat worms maintain the lengths of their telomeres they are immortal.

Chapter 14

TA-65: the only real "rejuvenation pill"

In chapter 13 we have seen that the length of the telomeres in the cell (cap at the ends of chromosomes, piece of plastic at the ends of a shoelace) determines the condition of the cell and thus our health and rate of aging.

We have seen that all body cells possess the latent capacity to lengthen the telomeres by activating the so-called Methuselah gene, the telomerase gene, which produces the miracle enzyme telomerase.

The 50.000 dollar question is: how do you activate the telomerase gene that lengthens your telomeres so that your life expectancy increases and the body becomes (partially) younger?

Thus far some 1000 telomerase activators have been found of which only one, TA-65, has been proven to be effective in man. Astragenol, another nutrient supplement has been shown (2013) to be moderately effective in in vitro (laboratory) tests.

The story of TA-65 is presented in the bestseller *The Immortality Edge,* by the leading expert in the field Dr. Michael Fossel and co-authors, from which I quote the following passage:

> **TA-65, for Those Who Want to Do It All**
> Ta-65, a nutritional supplement available through doctors licensed by T.A. Sciences, has huge potential to extend your life; that's the good news. The bad news is that it currently (2013) costs from twenty-two hundred to eight thousand dollars per year, depending on the dosage. There's good news, though, that will make the supplement much less costly, without losing its effectiveness. We spoke to Noel Thomas Patton, founder of T.A. Sciences, and

he told us [2010, J.G.D.]: "Long before *The Immortality Edge* is published we will have the peer-reviewed paper published by Dr. Calvin Harley that clearly demonstrates TA-65's effectiveness at lower doses than that which costs eight thousand dollars a year."

The lower doses, one that costs half of the current recommendation ($4000 and one that is one-quarter of the high-price tagged dose ($2,200 a year) are geared toward younger people (those who are just hitting their forties) and those whose budget precludes taking the more costly dose.

It may seem strange to put a price tag on your life, but we all do it every day without thinking about it. Every time we make a decision that affects our health and well-being based on what we can afford rather than what is best for us, we are putting a price tag on our lives. Before you object, consider how much money you spend on entertainment, eating out, and the like. For some people, this is yearly in excess of $2,400 to $8,000 dollars a year.

Keep that in mind as we describe the one and only proven telomerase activator that is available right now, in today's world: TA-65.

The TA-65 story begins in 2001. Hunting for a drug to treat chronic degenerative disease, Geron , then a small biopharmaceutical company in Menlo Park, California, began screening natural supplements that might target telomeres. After much trial and error, the Geron scientists discovered a single molecule in the astragalus plant (an ancient Chinese herbal medicine) that activates telomerase without any known toxicity. Because the company was more interested in finding ways to suppress telomerase in cancer cells, it licensed the rights to this molecule to a start up in New York City, T.A. Sciences Inc.

Beginning in 2002, T.A. Sciences spent five years testing and developing a highly concentrated form of astragalus, which it called TA-65. In 2005, the company was able to demonstrate through a double-blind, placebo-controlled study that people who took TA-65 showed marked improvement in measurable anti-aging biomarkers. Specifically, their immune systems were strengthened, some showed visual improvement, many showed increased sexual function, others reported that their energy levels rose, and skin elasticity improved for some (that is, they had younger looking skin).

Even more exciting is that in 2007, an independent company, Sierra Sciences in Reno, Nevada, was able to prove that TA-65 does indeed activate telomerase. Late studies conducted in Spain proved that TA-65 caused critically short telomeres to lengthen.

Because it is marketed as a supplement TA-65 needs no approval from the FDA. One implication of this is that T.A. Sciences cannot make any claims about TA-65's ability to prevent or cure diseases, even though there is probably a link between telomere length and age-related disease. TA-65 has been commercially available since 2007 without any reported adverse effects. Nevertheless, the following questions remain about the supplement:

- Does it cause cancer?
- Will it come down in price? (We have already answered that one - yes!)
- Has the government or any major university tested it?

The question of cancer is frequently asked because telomerase is activated to a high degree in about 85 percent of human cancers. Thus it is a natural concern that something that seems to mimic what cancer does might cause cancer. Although it is not 100 percent proven, it appears that the way that TA-65 activates telomerase is mild and far more natural than the huge and multiple ways that it is activated in cancer. That is, TA-65 is closer to the natural telomerase activation that appears in stem cells and germ-line cells than to the unbridled and ungoverned ways that telomerase is turned on in cancer. To date [2010], there are no studies linking

TA-65 use to cancer in any way. In fact, given the proven immune function benefits there are those who speculate that TA-65 provides more "good guys to fight cancer than bad guys."

The price tag is not likely to come down again anytime soon, because the proprietary process of extracting one specific molecule from the astragalus plant is complicated, and the molecule is only one of more than two thousand found in the plant. There are other astragalus-based supplements on the market that claim to activate telomerase, but tests have proven that they don't. These are much cheaper because they contain no TA-65 and because they don't actually activate telomerase [this is written in 2010, JGD].

Sierra Sciences has screened about 250,000 compounds and found 770 inducers. None of these is powerful enough to be used as a drug, but the search goes on. Assuming that Sierra Sciences is successful in finding the right compound, it will then take the company many years to go through all the stages of developing, testing, and marketing an FDA-approved drug. Current choices are therefore limited.

If you want to take a pill that will absolutely turn on telomerase, improve immune function, and has been shown to lengthen critically short telomeres, TA-65 is the only option for now. You can learn more about TA-65 and find a list of doctors who are licensed to prescribe it at the TA-Sciences Website, www.tasciences.com.

Chapter 15

L-Arginine: protection against atherosclerosis and heart attacks

The following report opened my eyes for the huge significance of the amino-acid L-arginine for atherosclerosis.

Dr. Joseph Prendergast, at the time cardiologist at Stanford University (Cal.) already had severe atherosclerosis in his abdominal arteries at the age of 17, as a CAT-scan requested because of vague abdominal symptoms, revealed. His father had his first severe heart attack at the age of forty-two. "You have the abdominal vessels of an 80-year old", the radiologist told him. Although he was symptom-free, he decided on the advice of Dr. Victor Dzau, director of Cardiovascular Research at Stanford, to take L-arginine to stop the progression of atherosclerosis. When years later another CAT-scan was taken the atherosclerosis had completely disappeared. In his own words:

"In 2001 I had another CAT-scan of my abdomen just as I had at the age of 37 when my atherosclerosis was discovered. The atherosclerosis was completely gone." A miracle! There is, except chelation therapy (see chapter 35) or Dr. Ornish' 'rabbit diet', nothing that can reverse atherosclerosis, when we leave vitamin C (chapter 16) out of consideration. What is the secret of arginine? The answer is simple: Nitric oxide, NO.

NO is present in smog, but also in your blood vessels and nervous tissue!

The medical use of NO began long ago, in the nineteenth century when Alfred Nobel was still alive. As you know Nobel was the inventor of dynamite. In the production of dynamite nitro-glycerine is used. The workers at the dynamite plants complained about headaches during working hours. At home the headache was gone. What was the cause? As was shown much later the dilatation of the blood vessels under the skull resulting from the released gas NO, nitric acid. In those days nitro-glycerine was already prescribed by doctors for angina pectoris. (pill under the tongue).

When Alfred Nobel suffered excruciating chest pains shortly before his death his doctors wanted to give him nitro-glycerine to alleviate the pain by dilating his coronary vessels. He obstinately refused, since it was unthinkable to him that an explosive could alleviate pain. Had he but listened he might have lived longer!

When Dr. Louis Ignarro presented his findings that the dilatation of blood vessels was caused by NO (chemically close to 'laughing gas') produced in the vessel wall, at a meeting held at the Mayo Clinic, the reaction was negative. Despite the hard evidence no-one would believe it. "You may have sniffed too much laughing gas (N2O)" a wag chimed in. Twelve years later, in 1998, Dr. Ignarro received the Nobel Prize for his ground-breaking discovery.

Nitro-glycerine produces vasodilatation by relaxing the smooth muscle tissue via NO but is unsuitable as a means for the treatment of narrowed arteries due to atherosclerosis. Incidentally, Viagra too, acts by releasing NO locally.

The ideal 'raw material' to strengthen the production of NO in the vessel wall in the long run is L-arginine, a natural amino acid that is present in food and that the body is able to manufacture.

The endothelium and atherosclerosis
As I said before, as a 'life-extender' you sometimes have to descend to the level of the cell in order to really *understand* and thus acquire the motivation to use a given supplement year in, year out.

The vessel wall is separated from the bloodstream by a kind of skin. This is called the endothelium and its constituent cells are correspondingly named endothelial cells. Endothelial cells play an important role in the formation of atherosclerosis, which, as you know, is characterized by a kind of gruel covered by a scab, the infamous *plaque*.

It is almost true to say that if the endothelium is strong and healthy you won't get atherosclerosis! Even existing atherosclerosis may disappear when the endothelium is restored to its healthy state, as the case of Dr. Prendergast illustrates.

Studies have shown that L-arginine activates the enzyme telomerase (chapter 13) via the local production of the gas NO, thus lengthening the telomeres of the endothelial cells, resulting in 'rejuvenation' of the endothelium. (Please read chapter 13 for a full explanation).

So, for your health it means that the 'normal' process of atherosclerosis can be slowed down or even reversed by the daily use of the supplement L-arginine.

Through this hugely important action of L-arginine – the production of NO gas in the endothelial cells - L-arginine supplementation (4-10 grams daily) offers the following benefits for your health according to the Nobel Prize winner professor Ignarro:

- lowers blood pressure
- improves circulation
- curbs the development of atherosclerosis
- reduces the risk of a heart attack
- reduces the risk of thrombosis and embolism (blood clots)

As professor Ignarro explains in his book *NO More Heart Disease,* atherosclerosis (and hypertension) are closely involved with the damage to the endothelium. The reduced production of NO leads to a vicious circle: more atherosclerosis (hypertension) → more damage to the endothelium → less NO → more atherosclerosis, etc.

Very significant is the fact that the production of NO decreases substantially after 40, resulting at 60 and over in a value less than half found in people at thirty and younger.[25]

---

25   This is determined by the giving of the vessel-dilating substance acetylcholine to test persons and measuring the blood flow in the underarm.

Atherosclerosis. The 'man in the street' would say when he hears this term, "Oh, no, I'm not demented, everything is still fine up here." Atherosclerosis is often wrongly associated with dementia, although you do can become demented if you are suffering from severe atherosclerosis.

Atherosclerosis is a 'normal' process that already starts at puberty ('yellow streaks' in the vessel wall, first found at autopsies of 19-year-old American soldiers during the Korean war).

Atherosclerosis – scale (junk) in the arteries - inexorably continues just as the calcification in your coffee machine when it has never been flushed with vinegar and is especially life-threatening in the elderly: well over half of the people die from the complications of atherosclerosis: stroke, heart attack, aneurysm, etc. Most thrombi are the result of an advanced state of atherosclerosis. It is no exaggeration to say that the two greatest threats to your health are atherosclerosis and cancer.

Cancer is a disease ('you either have it or you don't'), atherosclerosis is a time-dependent process that in some people progresses faster than in others.

If you got the wrong genes it progresses faster, as in the case of Dr. Prendergast; if you have hypertension or diabetes it also progresses faster as both high blood pressure and an elevated glucose level depress NO production and thus worsen the existing atherosclerosis.

Practical information for boosting your NO production
L-arginine is an amino-acid (building block of protein) that your body is able to produce. After forty this capacity declines. Via food the daily intake is on the average 5 gram L-arginine. For a detectable boosting of your 'normal' NO production in the endothelium at least 3 grams of L-arginine should be taken daily as supplement. The optimal amount is between 5 grams and 10 grams daily divided over three portions.

For best results it is recommended to combine this with the following supplements:

vitamin C 500 mg, vitamin E 200 mg, folic acid 800 mcg (microgram) and alpha lipoic acid 100 mg or less. A combination with the amino acid citrulline (200-1000 mg boosts the action of L-arginine. Citrulline can be obtained via internet, just like L-arginine, of course.

The NO production is boosted – apart from L-arginine – by nitrates and nitrites. The assertion that these substances cause cancer is wrong. The mere fact that your saliva contains these substances settles the issue.

Good sources of nitrates are spinach, broccoli, cauliflower and Brussels sprouts.
For the following reason these vegetables are *cardio-protective*: via the conversion of nitrate to nitrite in the mouth and in the stomach the production of NO in the endothelium is boosted.

Physical exercise, but also drinking a lot of water (5 glasses a day as recommended by Dr. Ignarro) enhances the production of NO.

The former explains why heart attacks often occur during sleep in the early morning hours. Then NO is at its lowest.

Warning. Arginine does not help with claudication (narrowing of the arteries in the legs). It is a preventive measure, not a 'cure'. Apart from stents, etc. only chelation therapy, a treatment developed by American cardiologists and internists in the fifties, is effective (see chapter 35).

The ABC of atherosclerosis
The distinctive feature of atherosclerosis is the plaque, a kind of pustule filled with gunge. The inner wall of a healthy artery when exposed looks as smooth as young skin. An atherosclerotic artery's inner wall looks like pockmarked skin, whereby the pocks are often fused together. The pustules protrude into the lumen leading to narrowing of the vessel.

When the endothelium is damaged certain cell types from the blood stream enter through the lining of the wall and accumulate in the underlying layer composed of smooth muscle cells. LDL (the 'bad' cholesterol) present in the vessel wall (the so-called 'intima') is then oxidized and 'swallowed up' by these emigrating cells, macrophages and others, causing them to swell up and assume a foamy appearance. This is why they are referred to as *foam cells*. These cells die on the spot, resulting in necrosis. Via inflammation factors smooth muscle cells are induced to multiply to form a non-malignant tumour. The end-result is 'gunk', atheroma (which means 'gruel') covered by a fibrous capsule. The term atherosclerosis obviously derives from 'atheroma'.

When the capsule bursts the (pro-clotting) contents of the plaque come into contact with the blood resulting in a thrombus that may close off the vessel. In the heart this will result in a cardiac infarction (heart attack). In the brain it results in a stroke, although the majority of strokes are the result of embolism from a calcified neck artery.

Atherosclerosis is just like hypertension: there are usually no symptoms until it is too late.

And almost everyone over sixty (including the teetotaller, vegetarian and non-smoker) has a risky degree of atherosclerosis at that age. With L-arginine you keep you endothelial cells in a healthy condition and thus decrease your future risk (*Always plan for the future, man!*). Dangerous cells like macrophages are unable to enter through healthy endothelium, whereby the process of atherosclerosis is stopped and recovery can begin. The most important factor in recovery is NO, discovered by Dr. Ignarro, better known as Dr. NO.

Chapter 16

Atherosclerosis: chronic subclinical 'scurvy'

In chapter 15 we have seen how we can protect ourselves against the underlying cause of strokes and heart attacks, the cause of death of the majority of people.

Are you afraid of atherosclerosis? No? Then you're not well informed, a fool, or just tired of living.

Knowledge is power. Just take your time, for this chapter may, with chapter 15, improve your life expectancy drastically. Even when you're still young: be prepared. What you're doing now or not doing may have far-reaching consequences for much later when you enter the 'danger zone'.

Make sure that atherosclerosis is kept at a minimum and you'll never have a stroke or heart attack.

Atherosclerosis is a chronic form of 'subclinical scurvy'
"What nonsense!" I can hear you think. This is the reaction of laymen but also of doctors. Very few doctors have ever heard of the scientific discipline 'evolutionary medicine'[26], which studies the evolutionary origin of certain diseases.

Atherosclerosis is a genetic condition, similar to, say, sickle cell anaemia (the red cells look like sickles instead of discs). This inborn form of anaemia is due to a mutation in the DNA that happened in the distant past in the malaria regions of Africa. As you may know a mutation is a (harmful) change in a gene. The important difference between atherosclerosis and sickle cell anaemia is

---

26 A good introduction is the book "EVOLUTIONARY MEDICINE", Rethinking the Origins of Disease' van Marc Lappé, Sierra Club Books.

that the latter occurs only in a small group of people while atherosclerosis is a genetic defect that affects all mankind.
What bullshit!
Just a little patience ...
All mammals, with the exception of man, big apes (primates) and the guinea pig produce their own ascorbic acid or vitamin C. (the term ascorbate is also used). All animals – from your cat to your goat - produce some 2-10 gram a day in terms of the body weight of man.

In animals - with the exception of apes and the guinea pig – atherosclerosis and myocardial infarction do not occur, except as a result of under function of the thyroid gland. As an illustration I mention a paper in the Journal of the American Veterinary Medical Assiociation (189, 227, 1986) in which (with difficulty) 21 dogs with atherosclerosis found at autopsy had been collected over a period of 14 years The cause was underactivity of the thyroid gland.

The reason for the absence of atherosclerosis in animals is that they produce ample amounts of vitamin C.

When the gene responsible for the manufacture of vitamin C (ascorbic acid) in the liver is experimentally switched off the test animal (dog, rat, etc.) develops atherosclerosis when given a vitamin C deficient diet. *Let me mention in passing that for most animals (dog, etc.) ascorbic acid is not a vitamin, for by definition a vitamin is a required molecule provided by the diet.*

The critical reader may wonder: if atherosclerosis is a subclinical form of scurvy why is there no bleeding? We all know that in the past sailors with scurvy suffered from bleeding gums, internal bleedings so-called *petechiae* as a result of weakening of the mortar of our tissues and blood vessels: connective tissue or collagen.

The reason is that in the course of the evolution our distant ancestors developed a 'putty' to seal off the weakened and leaky vessel wall.

Pauling's theory about the fundamental cause of atherosclerosis and coronary artery disease

Just by way of introduction: Linus Pauling is regarded as one of the greatest scientists of all time. In 1935 he published a book, *The Chemical Bond*, which transformed chemistry into a real science bases on quantum physics. Before that date chemistry was like an intricate game with empirical rules for smart puzzlers. He is the only scientist who earned two unshared Nobel prizes. When Pauling speaks the scientific community listens.

The essence of his theory (1989) is that atherosclerosis (the main cause of death) is due to chronic vitamin C deficit. It is a sub-clinical form of scurvy. Just like the self-sealing bike tire, which, when a puncture occurs, automatically seals it with silicones, so our body has 'learned' in the course of millions of years to seal the weakened vessel wall due to vitamin C deficit with a 'putty', a special form of LDH (the so-called 'bad cholesterol').

Atherosclerosis and vessel narrowing can be prevented by taking extra vitamin C (grams divided over the day) and the amino acid lysine that ensures that no excessive amounts of 'putty' are deposited in the vessel wall.

Of course the question is raised in your mind, "If Pauling's theory is correct, why have doctors not heard of it and why is it not generally applied in medicine?"

The answer is simple. Medicine is not a science but a business. Doctors are (without being aware of it) puppets manipulated by Big Pharma. Only patented drugs are prescribed for that's where the profits are. That's why the emphasis on statins, etc. in narrowed arteries and atherosclerosis (seen chapter 11). On Wiki's webpage 'Atherosclerosis' Pauling's theory is fully discussed.

A nice example. In the seventies scientists discovered that yoghurt (which contains lactic acid bacteria that are able to normalize the acidity of the vagina) is the most effective treatment of fluor alba (white discharge), a painful condition due to inflammation of the vagina. Numerous publications appeared in leading medical journals such as The American Journal of Gynaecology. Was this simple and effective treatment ever prescribed by doctors? *Forget it!*

There was no money to be made by Big Pharma, which through its sponsored symposia and drug salesmen are fully in charge.

The same holds for Pauling's therapy. There is not a penny to be made, so Pauling's theory and treatment is completely ignored by the medical community.

As has been shown scientifically via DNA mutations, some 30 million years ago or longer a mutation occurred, silencing the gene in our distant ancestor responsible for the production of ascorbate (vitamin C) in the liver. This ancestor was not a big ape but a tiny free-range animal. Don't forget: 30 million years ago was - in geological terms - only a short while after the disappearance of the dinosaurs 60 million years ago. The last common ancestor of man and gorilla lived 7 million years ago. Man originates, as you may know, from Africa. That is his 'home country', 'paradise lost'. The loss of the ability to produce ' ascorbate (vitamin C) was not a disaster, for our distant ancestors, just like the gorilla in the jungles of Africa, could find enough vitamin rich foods, making the risk of scurvy vanishingly small.

Some 100.000 (or 200.000) years ago the exodus of our ancestors began to other parts of the world, where glacial periods and drought led to a serious deficiency of vitamin C, resulting in scurvy. We know from the days before lemon was introduced that scurvy within months would lead to death from internal bleedings. The basic cause is that the body without vitamin C is unable to make strong connective tissue (collagen). In our body connective tissue is continually broken down and renewed.

Mortality among our emigrating ancestors must have been enormous and – scientifically speaking - we should regard it as a miracle that humanity survived.

What was our salvation?

In the course of thousands of years, via the Darwinian process of 'natural selection' and 'survival of the fittest', a mutation (in the DNA) occurred that enabled the body to make a kind of 'putty' that could stop the bleeding by sealing off the porous vessel wall.

This putty is (don't be alarmed) Lp(a), a substance closely related to the familiar LDL cholesterol, the 'bad' cholesterol. This did not result in the elimination of scurvy, but provided the body with a means to protect itself somewhat against the cause of death: massive bleedings.

The sailors of the seventeenth century also often died from bleedings despite Lp(a), the putty, which only confirms the fact that adhesives cannot always save a punctured tyre.

> Lp(a) is in fact a LDL–cholesterol particle surrounded by an adhesive layer. LDL-cholesterol is a hollow protein ball filled with cholesterol molecules. Lp(a) is this protein ball, enveloped by a sticky protein, apo(a), a kind of Velcro. Apo(a), the Velcro, seals of the holes, from an evolutionary view an elegant solution, especially because primitive man seldom reached the age of 40.
>
> Lp(a) and LDH deposition in the vessel wall lead however in the course of time to a chronic inflammation process in the vessel wall and thus to the development of the plaque, the pustule of atherosclerosis (see chapter 17).
>
> Atherosclerosis is nothing but an a pathological process on the basis of the evolutionary beneficial sealing with Lp(a) in the presence of vitamin C deficiency.

Let's have a closer look at the anatomy. We know that plaque (the 'pustule' of atherosclerosis) is not present everywhere in the arteries, but especially at locations where the vessel wall is most subject to overload, i.e. near the heart and in the coronary vessels. Stress factors are high blood pressure, turbulence and distortions of the arteries like in the beating heart. In the aorta blood pressure is at its highest while turbulence occurs at bifurcations, as in the neck arteries, the source of embolism and strokes.

Both high pressure (aorta) and distortions (coronary arteries) are important harmful causes. The situation is just like your garden hose where excessive water pressure and 'distortions' in the long run lead to cracks and tears.

The most putty is found where the most leaks occur: in and around the heart, so that's where the most atherosclerosis is found. In 1965 scientists showed that Lp(a) is exclusively deposited near cracks and tears.[27]

---

27 Lp(a) sticks to lysine in the vessel wall an amino acid which is a component of collagen and is set free when collagen disintegrates.

What is the solution?

In the first place making the vessel walls as strong as possible as to make them resistant to the stress of high pressure and distortions. This can be achieved only by improving both the quality and the quantity of the connective tissue (the so-called extracellular matrix) of the vessel wall: the job of vitamin C.

It is simple: just as in all mammals that produce their own vitamin C and thus never develop atherosclerosis we can prevent (the further development of) atherosclerosis by keeping the vessel wall of the arteries in optimal shape by vitamin C.

Practically this means that beside a healthy diet you should take at least three times a day a time-release coated tablet of 1000 mg vitamin C (or twice a day 1 sachet of 1000 mg liposomal vitamin C (see google)).

As treatment for atherosclerosis Pauling also recommends the amino acid lysine (3 gram/day as a powder or capsule divided over two portions). Due to this Lp(A) in the bloodstream binds to lysine in the blood instead of to the lysine threads in the damaged vessel wall.

Sherlock Holmes and Dr. Watson

A scientist is nothing but a Sherlock Holmes equipped with a microscope instead of a magnifier. Sherlock would propose a theory (about a murder, say) and aided by his faithful Dr. Watson he would then subject his theory to a critical analysis on the basis of available evidence.

Let's do something similar in the form of a critical question–and-answer game.

Question. If Pauling's theory is correct myocardial infarction does not occur in animals that produce their own ascorbate (vitamin C) since infarction is the result of narrowing of the coronary vessels due to atherosclerosis. Is this correct?

Answer. That's right; atherosclerosis and myocardial infarction (heart attack) are not found in animals that make their own ascorbate in the liver. Both your dog and the Hound of the Baskervilles in Conan Doyle's famous book do not get a heart attack. Petplace. com (*the web no 1 source of pet information*) states: "Myocardial infarction is rarely seen in a dog. The few cases of coronary artery narrowing found in dogs were associated with hormonal changes like decreased thyroid function."

Question. When animals that cannot produce vitamin C, like the guinea pig, are put on a vitamin C-deficient diet do they develop atherosclerosis as Pauling's theory predicts?

Answer. That's correct. The first study dates from as early as 1957 (G.C. Wallis, M.A.J .1, 77, 1957). When guinea pigs get scurvy as a result of extreme vitamin C deficiency they also develop atherosclerosis. No atherosclerosis was found in the control group. Since then scores of studies have confirmed this finding. It's worth mentioning that the plaques ('pustules') disappeared when vitamin C was given at an early stage.

Question. If Pauling's theory is correct in stating that humans have been saved by the 'natural selection' of 'putty' (a kind of LDL cholesterol) to protect the porous blood vessels during periods of vitamin C deficiency, then you would expect that this putty only occurs in man and (other) animals that are unable to produce vitamin C. Is this the case?

Answer. Correct. De 'putty' - the technical term is Lp(a) - is only found in species that are unable to make ascorbate: man, big apes, guinea pig and a few other tiny creatures.

Question. If Lp(a), the 'putty', is the cause of atherosclerosis you might expect Lp(a) to be present in the earliest stages of plaque formation. Has this been found?

Answer. That's correct. Lp(a) enters the vessel wall from the beginning. The earliest stage is identified at autopsy by so-called 'yellow streaks' and these are already present in all children over ten years old.[28]

No wonder, for we all suffer from chronic vitamin C deficiency (remember animals produce, in terms of human body weight, about 5 grams a day, while we get less than 100 mg in our food), so we are all in a 'pre-scurvy' stage. The 'yellow streaks' contain immune cells (so-called monocytes) laden with oxidized cholesterol, but the causative factor that starts the process is Lp(a), the putty against leakage in vitamin C deficiency.

Remark:
At autopsy Beisiegel found mainly Lp(a) in plaques rather than LDL cholesterol.

Question. If Pauling's theory is correct we should expect guinea pigs suffering from vitamin C deficiency to have elevated blood levels of the 'putty', Lp9A0. Is this the case?

Answer. That's correct. Pauling and Rath have shown that blood levels of Lp(a) are elevated in vitamin C deficient guinea pigs. An inverse relationship exists between the serum Lp(a) and serum vitamin C level.

Question. If Lp(a) exerts a causative role in coronary narrowing it should be an important risk factor for coronary heart disease and myocardial infarction. Is this the case?

Answer. That's right. A recent re-analysis of the famous Framingham epidemiological findings shows that Lp(a) is a ten times greater risk factor than LDL-cholesterol.

Question. If vitamin C deficiency is the cause of atherosclerosis one might expect that a high vitamin C-intake would greatly reduce the risk of myocardial infarction. Has this been found?

---

28 While LDL cholesterol is only harmful when oxidized and then digested by the so-called foam cells, Lp(a) is a causative factor at the earliest stage by binding to extracellular structures where it accumulates without being broken down (Beisiegel, U. *et. al*. European Heart Journal, 11 (SUPPL), 174).

Answer. Correct. In a study involving 11.400 individuals over a ten-year period is was found that people with the highest vitamin C intake had a 42 per cent lower risk of a heart attack than on average. This 'highest 'dose (1 gram) is still on the low side since animals without atherosclerosis (continually) produce 5-10 grams daily in terms of human weight.

We could continue for a while but I think Sherlock Holmes may by now have convinced both Dr. Watson and you, since none of the evidence falsifies Pauling's theory.

This should come as no surprise because Linus Pauling and Matthias Rath were granted the American patent for the treatment of coronary disease on the basis of Pauling's theory (US patent 5278189). The conditions for obtaining a US patent are very strict. One can only obtain a US patent when the invention (on the basis of the underlying theory) is fully supported by experimental findings and its efficacy demonstrated.

The daily application
Because atherosclerosis is the main cause of death and a source of a lot of health problems in later years while a deficit of Vitamin C is the basic cause, it is fully rational to take extra vitamin C besides a 'healthy diet'. How much? As stated above at least three times a day a time- release coated tablet (capsule) of one gram e.g. from Lamberts, which guarantees a 6-hour release. You could also take the so-called liposome-encapsulated vitamin C (see google) that can be taken twice a day.

I for one take 3 Lamberts coated tablets (1000mg), 1 sachet liposomal ascorbate and some 6 grams of vitamin C powder dissolved in grapefruit juice (sweetener added), taking little sips all day long. Of course vitamin C offers many other benefits as well (see also chapter 24).

Important note
The statement that taking high doses of vitamin C makes no sense because vitamin C is excreted in the urine when a dose of 200 mg or more is taken is (partially) correct when it refers to a single dose a day.

In view of this it is important to take vitamin C at regular intervals throughout the day in order to keep the blood level constant (and high). Remember, animals produce their ascorbate at a constant rate throughout the day.

One may compare the situation with a barrel with a hole at mid-height. When you fill it only once the water level never gets beyond the level of the hole. But if you fill it at a constant rate with a garden hose and the tap wide open the level gets higher despite the hole. This 'constant intake' throughout the day is called the *'dynamic flow model'*.

Actually the situation is far more complex, as I may illustrate with a personal anecdote. Before taking extra vitamin C I had frequent colds despite taking orange juice and following a healthy diet. I would need some twenty handkerchiefs a day and water would drip from my nose as from a leaky faucet. And, man, did I feel awful! I also had a bad skin with wide pores (pig's skin). After reading Pauling's book 'Vitamin C and the Common Cold' in 1973 I started taking vitamin C 1000 mg once a day. Ever since I don't have colds anymore and within months my skin had become normal (no more wide pores, etc.)

Lesson: despite taking 1000 mg only once daily, which according to the simplistic model makes no sense, the effect of taking a mega-dose was spectacular.

Lysine
If you are 60+, or already suffering from the clinical effects of atherosclerosis (coronary heart disease, etc.) I recommend you also take the amino acid lysine. As explained above it removes the deposit of the 'putty', Lp(a) from the vessel wall, resulting in a slow and steady reduction of existing atherosclerosis.

Personally I take 3 gram lysine divided over two portions daily. Of course lysine can be obtained via the internet.

Medical Appendix

Below I present a point by point discussion of Pauling's theory.

- Ascorbate deficiency is a first requirement for and the common characteristic of cardiovascular disease (CVD).

- Ascorbate deficiency results from the incapacity of man to produce ascorbate, combined with insufficient intake.

- The morphological consequences of chronic ascorbate deficiency are weakening of the connective tissue (in the vessel wall) and loss of endothelial barrier function.

- Thus, CVD is a form of pre-scurvy. The diversity of pathological mechanisms that lead to the clinical manifestation of CVD are primarily defence mechanisms directed toward stabilizing the vessel wall. After the loss of the endogenous ascorbate production in the course of evolution these defence mechanisms became life-saving. They counteracted the fatal consequences of blood loss via the scorbutic vessel wall.

- CVD is not found in animals that produce ascorbate.

- The main cause of the development of plaque is the deposition of Lp(a) in the ascorbate-deficient vessel wall.

- Experimentally it has been shown that every CVD patho-mechanism can be induced by ascorbate deficiency, including the formation of foam cells.

- In ascorbate-deficiency Lp(a) is selectively retained in the vessel wall. Apo(a), a component of Lp(a), neutralizes the increased permeability by compensating for collagen loss by binding to fibrin.

- Chronic lack of ascorbate leads to the accumulation of Lp(a) in the vessel wall. This results in the development of the plaque and CVD, especially in people with a genetically determined high level of Lp(A).

- Optimal intake of ascorbate prevents the development of CVD. Ascorbate reduces existing plaques and thus lowers the risk of heart attack and stroke.

Chapter 17

Atherosclerosis: the 'silent killer'

It is sometimes said that hypertension is the 'silent killer', because people with high blood pressure live on the average ten years less.

'Silent' because there are no symptoms and then - out of the blue - a stroke or heart attack. But while ten per cent of the elderly suffer from hypertension virtually everyone above 50 has a potentially life threatening degree of atherosclerosis.

By the way: hypertension is dangerous not because of the high pressure itself but because it accelerates de development of atherosclerosis.

Because atherosclerosis is the major cause of heart attacks and strokes it is of importance to gain a clear understanding of the nature of the silent threat to your health and life.

In the foregoing chapter we have seen that the fundamental cause of atherosclerosis is a chronic vitamin C deficiency and that vitamin C supplementation offers the best prevention and protection.

But when this process, which starts at puberty, further develops in the course of decennia the situation becomes both pathologically as well as therapeutically much more complex since by then the picture is a lot more complicated than just the accumulation of Lp(a), the special form of the bad cholesterol, LDL cholesterol.

Next I'll present a picture of the pathology of atherosclerosis and its fingerprint, the plaque.

Healthy artery and 2 stages of atherosclerosis

Atherosclerosis: the picture
Just as sickle cell anaemia constitutes a genetic disease of the blood, as we have seen in chapter 16, so atherosclerosis is a genetic disease of the artery wall. Although the beginning is simple, the final result is complex.

As we have seen in chapter 16 it starts with the deposition of Lp(a) and LDL cholesterol in the vessel wall. This leads to an invasion of special white blood cells from the immune system: so-called monocytes (don't get put off by unfamiliar names) invade through the one cell thick layer 'skin' of the vessel, the endothelium, and literally swallow up the meanwhile oxidized cholesterol molecules. Since these monocytes packed with cholesterol look like foam–filled cells under the microscope they are aptly called 'foam cells'.

In this manner a process is initiated which is in effect a chronic inflammation. In inflammation infection may be involved but this is often not the case at all, like here.

When you step on a rusty nail inflammation results, characterized by pain, redness, heat and swelling, but chronic inflammation is mostly a silent insidious process whereby, like in other forms of inflammation, white blood cells and other components of the immune system are involved.

According to current opinion atherosclerosis is regarded as inflammation.

I will not bother you with the very complex details of the fully developed plaque, the 'pustule' of atherosclerosis.

But it is of some importance to point out that two forms of plaques are clinically distinguished: the 'classical' plaque characterized by a hard cortex and a pulpy content ('athero'=gruel), which accounts for the name atherosclerosis. This plague protrudes into the lumen and is (thus) the cause of blood vessel narrowing.

The other type of plaque looks very harmless at first sight. It is aptly called, "the soft vulnerable plaque" and constitutes the main cause of the much-feared myocardial infarction (heart attack).

In the early nineties pathologists at Harvard University had found that the cause of the infarction was not located at the stricture due to a large protruding plaque, but that the (obstructing) thrombus was at the site of a small, level plaque, the "soft, vulnerable plaque". Further studies showed that this was the main culprit. This small level plaque has a thin vulnerable cortex. When a crack occurs (usually from enzymatic action from within) blood comes into contact with the mushy contents of the plaque. This contents does not act like an anticoagulant but as a pro-coagulant, initiating coagulation. The result is a thrombus that obstructs the artery in seconds: myocardial infarction.

This soft vulnerable plaque cannot be seen by angiography and so is literally a 'ticking time bomb'. Only by intensive vitamin C and L- arginine supplementation (see previous chapters) and chelation therapy (chapter 35) an existing soft vulnerable plaque can be eliminated, or, more correctly, may be expected to have been cleared.

Personal note: This is one reason why I have been taking chelation therapy (EDTA infusions,) for over thirty years now: to keep my coronary arteries clean and so my heart beating.

At a later stage the classical plaque becomes calcified. The extent of calcification of the coronary arteries is determined by a CT-scan and is expressed by the so-called calcium-score. A value greater than 50 means 'danger'. The calcium score is lowered by chelation therapy (chapter 35), which removes calcium from the vessel wall and shrinks existing plaques.

But whether the infarction results from a protruding plaque or a thrombus resulting from a fractured soft vulnerable plaque, the fundamental cause is the same: atherosclerosis.

How to combat advanced atherosclerosis?

One way is to reduce inflammation.

Statins have been shown to reduce the inflammation in the vessel wall, an action wholly independent from that on cholesterol. But in view of the many side-effects of statins (see chapter 11) their use to

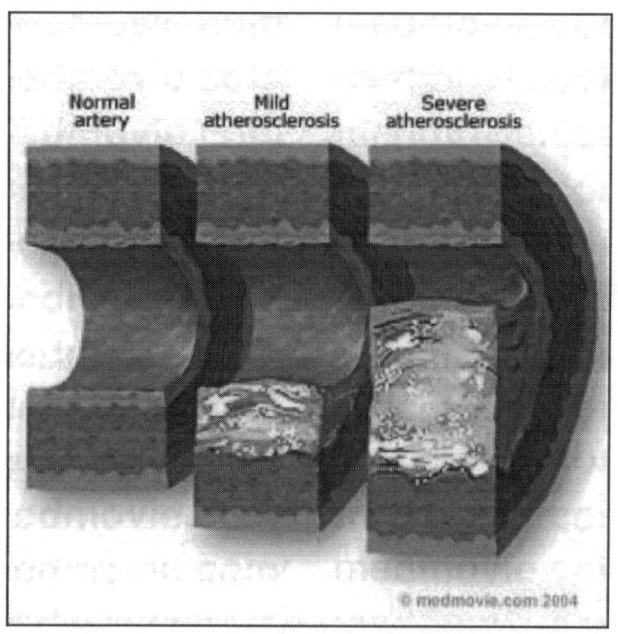

protect against heart attacks cannot be recommended. In over twenty studies only one (the so-called ASTEROID–study) has shown a regression of atherosclerosis by statins. Moreover, the effect was minor.

The most effective way to 'clean' narrowed coronary arteries (angina pectoris) is chelation therapy, whose efficacy has been confirmed by the gold-standard: a double-blind crossover statistical study (TACT study) in 2013 (see chapter 35).

The usual treatment of coronary heart disease is medicinal: statins, aspirin, beta-blockers, ACE-inhibitors, calcium-blockers) or surgical (bypass, stent). Bypass or stents do not improve life expectancy. This is acknowledged by Paul Biolette, vice-president of Boston Scientific, a leading producer of stents who declared: "It's really not about preventing heart attacks per se; the obvious purpose of the procedure is palliation and symptom relief. "

That makes sense, because atherosclerosis is not a 'plumber's problem 'but a systemic disease of the coronary vessels.

With the exception of vitamin C and arginine supplementation as well as chelation therapy (developed by American cardiologists and in 1960 given the FDA approval 'effective against atherosclerosis') the treatment of atherosclerosis is sadly ineffective.

For the sake of completeness I'll mention some common non–medicinal measures (see google for more information):

- Niacin (vitamin B3) in high doses. The unpleasant side–effect is hot flushes.
- A low-cholesterol diet. Not very effective because the body produces some 80 per cent of the total cholesterol and tends to increase production when on a low-cholesterol diet. Moreover cholesterol plays only a minor role in atherosclerosis (see previous chapters).
- The avenanthramids in oatmeal exert a favourable influence by reducing inflammation in the vessel wall.
- Omega-3 (fish oil) supplementation has been shown to be effective in six double-blind clinical studies. This is achieved by reducing inflammation.
- The action of homocystein-inhibitors such as vitamin B6, B12 and folic acid is minor.

I would like to end this brief survey by quoting a passage from Wikipedia on atherosclerosis. How authoritative is Wikipedia? A study published in the leading scientific journal *Nature* showed that the articles in Wikipedia contained fewer errors than those in the famed Encyclopaedia Britannica. A Wiki-article (without 'warning sign') can be regarded as authoritative.

The scale of vitamin C benefits on the cardiovascular system led several authors to theorize that vitamin C deficiency is the primary cause of cardiovascular disease. The theory was unified by twice Nobel Prize winner Linus Pauling and Matthias Rath. They point out that vitamin C is produced by almost all animals, with few exceptions, including mankind and the great apes. This is due to a genetic deficiency that arose with the common ancestor of humans and apes. To survive humans and apes must eat sufficient vitamin C. Without vitamin C humans develop scurvy. Vitamin C is an essential element in insuring that the vascular system is strong and flexible. Pauling and Rath suggest that a deficiency causes weakness in the arterial system and the body compensates by trying to stiffen the artery walls using common blood elements [Lp(a)], see chapter 16]. This causes the effect known as atherosclerosis. They suggest that manifestations of cardiovascular diseases are merely overshoot of body defence mechanisms that are involved in stabilization of vascular wall after it is weakened by the vitamin C deficiency and the subsequent collagen degradation.

The Unified Theory of Human Cardio Vascular Disease suggests that atherosclerosis may be reversed and cured, but there has been no testing or trial of Pauling's vitamin C theory.

It figures, for who will fund it? A double-blind study costs tens of millions of dollars and neither BIG PHARMA nor cardiologists are in the least interested in proving Pauling right. For BIG PHARMA it would be an enormous loss of income and cardiologists would be digging their own grave professionally since the most effective 'medicine' would not need a prescription and coronary patients would, like your dog, be conspicuous by their absence.

Immoral? No, only all too human. Bernard Shaw's famous dictum "All professions are conspiracies against the laity" holds, as I can testify as an insider, for the medical profession in particular!

Although the definitive scientific proof is still lacking there are strong statistical indications confirming the correctness of Pauling's theory, as discussed in chapter 16. In a 10-year survey involving more than 10,000 subjects it was found that those who had the highest intake of vitamin C had a 42 percent lower risk of a heart attack than on the average. And, mind you, here the highest daily dose was still a moderate one with regard to the protection of the blood vessels: one gram a day. And remember, the evidence presented in the Sherlock Holmes and Dr Watson exchange (chapter 16) fully supports Pauling's theory, which for the unbiased observer should be no longer in doubt.

Chapter 18

Exercise and its benefits

This is one of the shortest chapters of this book. Why? Because for me the material is tedious to write about. It is as simple as that.

In the seventies and the eighties everybody was jogging. For jogging was a MUST, according to the health gurus.

Times have changed, statistics have improved.

It is now well established that just walking three hours a week or cycling 2 hours a week is sufficient to protect the body over time against many aging diseases and conditions and improve your life expectancy. A Harvard paper mentions the following benefits:

- Improves your chances to live longer and healthier.
- Helps to protect you against heart problems, strokes and TIA's, hypertension and undesirable lipid-patterns [cholesterol, etc.].
- Helps to protect you against certain cancers, including colon cancer and breast cancer.
- Helps to prevent diabetes (type 2).
- Helps to prevent osteoporosis [especially walking, J.G.D.].

The immediate benefits are also worthwhile:

- Prevents weight gain.
- Improves cardiac and pulmonary function.
- Improves sleep.

It should be emphasised that 3 hours walking a week or two hours cycling is sufficient to obtain these positive results.

You may divide this over the week, like walking daily for half an hour or cycling for 20 minutes.

Chapter 19

Estrogen replacement after the menopause?

In the nineties and before many gynaecologists, general practitioners and anti-aging doctors prescribed long-term estrogen therapy for slowing down the process of aging (inclusive skin, vagina, etc.) under the motto "Feminine for ever" and to prevent osteoporosis and other aspects of lack of estrogen, the female hormone produced by the ovaries.

A female nurse who had worked in old people's homes for many years once told me, "Elderly women are generally more '*defeminized*' than elderly men are '*demasculinized*'. Elderly women are 'neutral beings' in contrast to elderly men." An astute observation. This is due to the fact that the production of sex hormones abruptly falls to near zero in the menopause while that of the male gradually declines but never reaches zero. This difference is particularly evident in the bones: the extent of osteoporosis in elderly women is far greater than in elderly men.

Sometimes it makes sense to pause at a truism.
"What is the most important organ of women?"
"The uterus."
"Wrong, the ovaries. Without ovaries, no pregnancy, no 'woman', but a 'neutral' person with poor health, premature aging and reduced life expectancy.
We can learn a lot from the biological consequences of removal of the ovaries at a younger age, i.e. in the 'fertile period' (20-40 years).

This equates to a premature menopause because of the loss of female hormones produced by the ovaries.

In every textbook and on the internet (enter: ovariotomy) you will find the following list of harmful medical effects:

1. early death (lower life expectancy)
2. cardiovascular diseases
3. stroke
4. early dementia
5. osteoporosis
6. Parkinson disease

Moreover it results in premature and accelerated aging, diminished sexual function (libido, orgasm, vaginal dryness, etc.) depression, anxiety symptoms and cognitive defects (poor memory, poor concentration, etc.).

Conclusion
The early, artificially induced, hormonal menopause teaches us that the loss of sex hormones (estrogens) has very serious consequences for your health, life expectancy and aging.

It has been shown by the 30-years *Mayo Clinic Study on Oophorectomie and Aging* that the most serious effects only become clinically manifest after 15 years.

One of the most striking consequences of loss of estrogen is accelerated osteoporosis. The incidence of osteoporosis is five times higher in women than in men. The reason? Testosterone production is sufficiently maintained in elderly men, while in women the production of sex hormones (estrogens) stops after around 50.

As stated earlier the sex hormones (testosterone and estrogen) constitute the best natural protection against osteoporosis (brittle bones).

Although osteoporosis is, e.g. like hypertension, a 'silent' disease, its consequences in the longer term are profound. Loss of height (shrinking), the well-known *douarière hump* (collapse of neck vertebrae) and the much feared hip fracture after 70, resulting in 15 percent of women dying of pulmonary complications within weeks, as well as chronic debilitating low back pains are the most conspicuous outcomes.

Why is studying the artificial menopause at a younger age relevant to 50+ women? Simply, because there is a lot of reference material, while there is none in women after 50-odd: everybody is hormonally deficient, so, the accelerated aging due to loss of estrogens is simply attributed to 'normal aging' by doctors.

Before the turn of the century estrogen replacement therapy was widely applied by gynaecologists, GP's and anti-aging doctors to prevent osteoporosis and other undesirable consequences of lack of estrogen (see above).

In 2002 the findings of a large American study suggested that the long term use of estrogens substantially increases the risk of breast cancer.

Confusion and consternation among doctors, dismay among women. The sale of these hormones dropped by more than 50 percent, because doctors only prescribed estrogen for hot flushes, etc. Since 2002 this mantra holds: "**No estrogens after the menopause because of cancer risk**". End of the story.

Studies carried out between 2003 and 2013 showed that this conclusion was both premature and wrong. To give you an early idea: the risk of breast cancer with the use of so-called bio-identical hormones (natural hormones produced by human ovaries) is no higher than with the consumption of 2 glasses of wine a day, that is, at the most, 20 percent higher. (This may seem 'much', but isn't, see below).

Against this minimal risk are the enormous benefits of correcting the 'hormonal castration' in the menopause, i.e. neutralizing (see list above):

- early death
- cardiovascular diseases
- increased risk of stroke
- increased risk of dementia

- osteoporosis
- Parkinson's disease

and, what many women treasure: the benefit of staying **'feminine forever'**.

Breast cancer risk factors: estrogen too?
As an introduction to a better understanding let me begin with a brief discussion of breast cancer risk factors.

What is the greatest risk factor of breast cancer?

Being a woman. Women have a risk of getting breast cancer during their lifetime of 1 in 8 (in the Netherlands and elsewhere in the West). So, in a manner of speech, when you have 8 women in a room 1 will get breast cancer.

How about men? During their lifetime the risk is 1 in 1000, so, more than 100 times less. What distinguishes a woman from a man? The sex gland that produces the sex hormones.

Does this mean that de sex gland (ovary, testis) is the cause of this enormous difference in risk?

Until fairly recently it was thought that the difference in sex hormones was the one and only factor for de difference between male and female.

This is not the case. As you know the difference is in the chromosomes. As you have been taught in school, the mother provides at conception an X-chromosome and the father either a X-chromosome or a Y-chromosome. When the embryo is XY it is a boy and in the case of XX it is a girl.

The Y-chromosome contains all the genetic information for the creation of a male while the 'extra' X-chromosome of a girl (embryo) contains all the genetic information for being female (although, by the way, only 10 percent of the DNA in this chromosome is utilized for this purpose).

'Being female' is thus determined by this 'extra' X-chromosome, which also contains the genetic information for the female hormones.

But – and this is the message - being female is determined by the 'female genes', among which the genes for the female hormones play a minor role.
The greatest risk of breast cancer is being a woman (not estrogens).

In comparison to the risk of the average fertile woman this risk is increased by a number of factors.
In order to offer you an idea of relative risk of taking estrogens the table below is presented (explanation: for example 4 means a 4 times greater risk than normal (400 %).

Table:

BRCA mutation (genetic)	>	5
Early menarche (first menstruation)		2
Late menopause		1.7
The "Pill"		1.25
late pregnancy		2
Overweight	>	1.5
'Sedentary'		1.5
alcohol		1.5
advanced age	>	5

For the discussion of the extra risk of breast cancer with the use of estrogens this table is most illustrative. Why?
Because different studies on estrogens related to breast cancer show a risk varying between 0.8 (20 percent protection) and 1.3 (30 percent extra risk).

When you study the list you may wonder, "What the heck are we talking about?"
Social drinking (let's say 4 glasses of wine a day) presents a risk of 1.5 (50 per cent extra risk, which may seem a lot, but is not in

absolute numbers), the use of the contraceptive pill, 1.25, lack of exercise, 1.5, overweight, greater than 1.5, etc.

On the basis of these numbers – even if estrogen would increase the risk by 1.3 - there is no need for consternation or dismay.

1.3 is about equal to the risk of using the Pill and lower than the risk of social drinking.

It is worth mentioning that you can needlessly scare people (laymen) to death with the clever use of statistics (as shown in chapter 11).

Let me illustrate. If within a given period (say, one year) 11 out of 1000 women get breast cancer, then, when the risk factor is 1.2 say, this means that instead of 11, 13 out of 1000 women will get it. This looks quite a bit less alarming than the number 1.2.

You will get an even clearer picture by realizing that instead of 989 per 1000 women, 987 stay healthy! "What are we talking about, peanuts?" you may wonder. Since the end of Wold War II scientists have carefully studied the possible link between estrogen use and the risk of breast cancer. In 1963 (more than 50 years ago) the editorial board of the authoritative *Yearbook of Cancer* concluded, "… that there is not a single case in the literature of estrogen inducing cancer." The quest has continued with unflagging zeal ever since, but it should be clear by now that it is a matter of splitting hairs.

This is not a trivial matter, but as we'll see, these hairs are few in number or absent altogether, dependant on the nature of the estrogen therapy provided.

This leads us to the next question: "What is estrogen therapy?"

The replacement of the missing hormone estradiol in the (post) menopause can strictly speaking only be realized by the administration of the (bio-identical) hormone estradiol. This sounds logical, but in medical practice synthetic hormones or animal hormones with a different chemical structure are often prescribed: ethinylestradiol and Premarin (trade name) respectively. The latter is derived from the urine of pregnant mares.

Estrogen Replacement Therapy (**ERT**) is by definition only possible with bio-identical female hormones, of which estradiol is the most important.

So, **ERT** is estradiol therapy (often, for 'technical reasons', supplemented with the natural hormone progesterone).

All other estrogen treatments are not **ERT**, but **ET** (estrogen therapy)

ET after the menopause is fine, but it is not **ERT**, the gold standard for the replacement of the missing hormones in the (post)menopause.

Why dwell on this distinction, you may wonder?

Because studies that found a significant increase in cancer risk (1.3) refer to **ET** and not to **ERT**.

This doctor and other anti-aging physicians emphatically advise **ERT** rather than **ET**, i.e. the use of the bio-identical hormone estradiol.

More generally a distinction is made between Hormone Replacement Therapy (**HRT**) and Hormone Therapy (**HT**). Only natural human hormones qualify for HRT.

Let me reveal the final conclusion at this early stage: long-term estradiol treatment does not increase the risk of breast cancer.

But I'm running ahead of my story.

The breast cancer scare

Just as the misconception that the use of testosterone increases the risk of prostate cancer (see chapter 20) has its roots in a worthless study in a distant past, so the medical mantra "estrogen causes breast cancer" is historically based on invalid research on mice in the fifties.

To offer you a historical glimpse let me quote from my own paper published in the Dutch Journal of Medicine (title translated) from 1966 (110, 1270), presented in simplified form.

"In general cancer can only be induced by giving fantastically high doses of estrogen to mice with a strong genetic predisposition to cancer. High doses given to 'normal' mice failed to cause cancer, while normal ('physiological') doses of estrogen were unable to cause cancer in cancer-sensitive mice.

In higher animals estrogen, even when given in enormous doses, does not cause breast cancer or other cancers. In particular all attempts to cause cancer in apes by giving staggering amounts of estrogen have failed."

What has been retained in the collective subconscious memory of the medical community?
Cancer inducement by administering staggeringly high doses estrogen to highly cancer-susceptible mice!
This makes sense, for a positive result (cancer) is also in the collective memory better conserved than negative results (no cancer in normal mice).

In the course of time this result has been condensed to the fallacy, "**Estrogens cause cancer in mice.**"

An absurdity, but medicine is full of absurdities, among which the mantra of the cardiologists, "No more than three eggs a week", of the urologists, "Testosterone causes prostate cancer" and of the gynaecologists, "Estrogens cause breast cancer".

A medical mantra repeated by generations of doctors, eventually becomes a truism.

Driven by this 'truism' many gynaecologists have since the fifties raised a warning finger against the long-term use of estrogen in the (post)menopause without a shred of statistical evidence.

That belief and facts may be at odds for even the most fervent supporters of the cancer hypothesis is illustrated by the following quote from the book *Gynaecologic Cancer* (1956) by Dr. Corsaden a fervent adherent of the cancer theory, "In humans there is suggestive but not positive evidence that estrogens have caused cancer in the female breast."

Nearly 35 years later the situation was still the same.

In 1992 an editorial article in the Dutch Journal of Medicine entitled "Estrogen replacement therapy after the menopause and the risk of breast cancer" declared, *"Generally, estrogen replacement is considered safe with respect to the risk of breast cancer."*

"Estrogen and breast cancer". Old wives' tales, scare mongering? Here too the well-executed statistical study has the final word, despite the fact that in test animals the administration of estrogen in normal doses does not cause breast cancer or other forms of cancer.

Till 2002 the results of various studies oscillated between 1.2 and 0.8, or, 20 percent extra risk or rather 20 percent protection. More concretely: instead of 10 out of 1000 women getting breast cancer each year either 12 or 8 out of 1000 estrogen–treated women would get breast cancer. This result is acceptable and (in the worst scenario) is no higher than the extra risk of drinking two glasses of wine daily or using the contraceptive pill (see above).

In fact, fully justified in view of the enormous benefits of estrogen replacement in the menopause.

In 2002 a bombshell was thrown by an article in the JAMA (Journal of the American Medical Association)

The large-scale *WHI (Women's Health Initiative) study* showed a breast cancer risk of 26 percent: 26 instead of 20 percent or minus 20 percent obtained by earlier studies.

This result, widely reported by the media, resulted (as mentioned above) in consternation among doctors and panic among women. In one blow estrogen replacement therapy lost its appeal.[29]

Closer analysis (2009) of the data even showed a much higher risk, i.e. 100 percent greater risk of breast cancer (value 2.0). So, 20 out of 1000 women in one year instead of 10.

This result was also obtained in the British *One Million Women Study* that appeared in 2003 in the leading medical journal *The Lancet*.

100 percent extra risk, equal to the extra risk of a woman whose sister has earlier been diagnosed with breast cancer. Totally unacceptable!

---

29 NEJM, 368, 573, 2009.

This shocking result however does not refer to HRT (Hormone Replacement Therapy), but to HT (Hormone Therapy), or, more specifically, not to ERT (Estrogen Replacement Therapy), but to ET (Estrogen Therapy).

For Estrogen Replacement Therapy (i.e. with bio-identical hormones) this result is totally irrelevant.

Moreover, the findings refer to the **combined use of an estrogen and a progestin (artificial analogue of progesterone), the so-called combination therapy** and not to the use of the bio-identical hormone, estradiol, in isolation. It was later shown that the progestin was the main culprit. What is a progestin? It is, as stated earlier, a synthetic variant of the natural 'pregnancy hormone' progesterone that is produced by the ovaries in de second half of the menstrual cycle.

Before we proceed a brief explanation is in order. Wrongly, most doctors believe that in order to prevent an increased risk of uterus cancer, it is necessary to give a woman besides estrogen either the natural pregnancy hormone progesterone or a progestin during part or most of the cycle to make sure that the uterus mucous membrane does not become too thick (hypertrophy), resulting in an increased risk of uterus cancer.

It is in fact sufficient to give progesterone (progestin) only three or four times a year for 2 weeks in order to prevent this thickening (hypertrophy).

The bottom line is that most doctors provide the combination therapy (estrogen plus progestin) instead of monotherapy: only estrogen.

The fore-mentioned *Women's Health Initiative Study* covers the combination preparation Prempro (the inquisitive reader may want to know that this preparation contains besides estrogens from pregnant horses the progestin medroxyprogesterone).

Later studies showed that the progestin in Prempro and other combination preparation was the culprit.

The pharmaceutical giant Pfizer who took over Prempro's producer Wyeth in 2009, has thus far (Bloomberg) (2014) paid about one billion dollars in settlements of lawsuits filed on behalf of six thousand breast cancer victims from long-term use of Prempro. Peanuts for Pfizer!

In passing it may be mentioned that Wyeth with its two hormone preparations Premarin (that contains horse estrogens) and Prempro has a near monopoly position in the United States. Prior to 2012 fifteen million women in the USA used Prempro, which represents a turnover of three billion dollars.

The sponsor of the WHI study was the NIH (National Institutes of Health).

In a 2004 NIH report Dr. B. Alving, the leading investigator of the WHI study, stated that monotherapy (only estrogen) – quote- *"has not increased the risk of breast cancer during the time of study."* (6 years).

In other words, also in the earth shaking WHI study it was shown that the use of estrogen-only (monotherapy) does not increase the risk of breast cancer.

As an encore, it turned out that it even reduced the risk of colon cancer by 30 percent.

Superfluously this conclusion was confirmed by professor M. Stefanick in a statistical re-analysis of the WHI study which appeared in the leading medical journal *New England Journal of Medicine* (*NEJM, 360, 573, 2009*).

With this the question of whether or not ERT, because of breast cancer risk, has in fact been resolved. Provided administered correctly ERT (estradiol replacement therapy) is completely safe.

This conclusion has also been corroborated by other - well-conducted studies - ('randomised', etc.). In order not to burden you unduly I'll mention only two recent studies.

On the basis of a randomized double-blind study the *Australian National Health and Research Council declared in 2005* in a circular to doctors, "*Estrogen-only therapy has little or no effect on breast cancer incidence.*"

Even more positive is the report in the *International Herald tribune* and *The New York Times* (1-4-2011) which states that "*Women who had used estrogen alone had a 23 per cent lower risk of breast cancer compared with those who had taken a placebo.*"

This conclusion is again corroborated by an analysis of the *WHI* estrogen–only group that appeared in *Lancet Oncology* in 2012 (Anderson, G.L. et.al. March 2012). Compared to the placebo group women from the estrogen-only group had a lower risk to develop breast cancer and a lower risk to die from it.

To wind up the discussion one more observation.

Since ERT in the menopause does not involve only giving estradiol (estrogen only), but also the periodic addition of progesterone (the natural pregnancy hormone) to protect the uterus (see above) it is of importance to evaluate the breast cancer risk of the combination estradiol and progesterone.

A well-conducted long-term French study involving 80.000 women (Fournier, A. et.al., Breast Cancer Res Treat,107, 193, 2008) showed that the combination estradiol-progesterone (note: not the synthetic progestin, but the natural hormone), even when given monthly, has a relative risk of 1.0, that is, no increase of breast cancer risk whatsoever.

Final conclusion
It is certain that estradiol replacement therapy in the menopause with periodic addition of progesterone (3-4 times a year), does not increase the risk of breast cancer and even with high probability lowers the risk.

To wind up the argument I present the following 'philosophical consideration', a deep one. If estrogens would be an important factor in the causation of breast cancer one would expect that breast cancer occurs less often after the menopause (no estrogen) than during the fertile period (plenty of estrogen).

Nothing is further from the truth. According to a Canadian study (2005) the *incidence* (here defined as the number of new cases per 100.000 within 10 years) between 30 and 39 is 850 and between 50 and 59 6000. An difference of 700 percent.

The most important factor in breast cancer is age. Just like with all cancers: the older the person the greater risk of breast cancer. (See also the table above, which shows a 500 percent increase or greater.

Practical tips
Just as in the case of the contraceptive pill YOU, not your doctor, are in charge. If your doctor refuses to cooperate show him this chapter or find another doctor.

Avoid combination preparations with continuous estrogens and progestins such as Acivelle, Climodien, Femoston continu and Kliogest.

It is best to use an estrogen-only preparation such as Progynova, Premarin, Zumenon, Dagynil or plasters: Estradiol plasters (Sandoz), Dermistil and Climara.

When an estrogen-only preparation is used, then 3 or 4 times a year progesterone or a progestin should be added to keep the uterus mucous membrane thin. But every physician is familiar with this.

If desired you may use a combination preparation, whereby progestin is only present in the second half of the cycle (10 to 14 days, instead of 28 days).

Examples are: Trisequens, Premarin Plus, Femeston and Climene.

It all sounds a bit complicated, but consider this passage a reference text. Good luck!

This doctor's first choice is a plaster: Estradiol plasters (contain estradiol) for 3 months. In the 4th month oral progesterone (Progestan) is added for two weeks, resulting in a menstruation (shedding of mucous membrane).

Warning
In the instruction leaflet of all estrogen preparations (both synthetic and natural) you will find a warning of a slightly higher risk of breast cancer. Although natural estrogens (estradiol) offer 'protection', it makes sense from the point of view of the producer to mention this *caviat,* since in a lawsuit the voice of the 'expert' - most often a professor - is decisive, even if he/she is not familiar with the latest scientific findings, such as those discussed above. For the judge the opinion of the 'expert' is the deciding factor.

Note
There are a number of 'schemes' for prescribing estrogen replacement. In my medical practice a favourite scheme is the following.

In order to prevent the risk of undue 'thickening' of the uterus (called hypertrophy or hyperplasia) progesterone or a progestin should be given periodically (see above).

For this I prescribe the natural hormone progesterone (Progestan or Utrogestan) and copy nature's rhythm: a 'stop-week'.

Four times a year in the last week of the three week hormone cycle (that is, before the 'stop week') progesterone is added.

So, during this last week the patient receives both estrogen (estradiol) and progesterone. During the stop-week menstruation may occur.

Even when this is not the case the uterus mucosa has shrunk.

Alternatively, progesterone may be given during the last 12 days of the 3-week hormone cycle. Then menstruation is (nearly always) assured.

General rule: in case you, for some reason, do not tolerate estrogen replacement, you may lower the dose or stop altogether.

Chapter 19A

May women who have had breast cancer take estrogen (ERT)?

This chapter is meant for women who have had breast cancer and have been 'cured'. Studying chapter 19 is a prerequisite for a sound understanding of the content of this chapter.

The general guideline is that because of the danger of the recurrence of the disease the use of estrogen is contra-indicated in women who have had breast cancer.

This is the conventional wisdom, but is it true?

As early as 2001 this view was questioned in the Netherlands on the basis of an Australian study that appeared in the *Journal of the National Cancer Institute* (O'Meary et.al. 93, 754, 2001).

In the *Dutch Journal of Medicine* (2001, 145, 2202) Dr. J. Mamerlynck wrote in a paper under the heading, **Perhaps postmenopausal hormone replacement is not at all contra-indicated after breast cancer:**

"Hormonal Replacement Therapy (HRT) is considered 'contra-indicated' in women who had been treated in the past for breast cancer. For, estrogens have proliferating effects [cell division promoting] on breast tissue and play a still poorly understood role in the causation of breast cancer. These detrimental effects of exogenous estrogens [administered estrogens] have however never been proven and are therefore questioned."

After a discussion of the results of the O'Meary study the Dutch author confirms the conclusion of the Australian study. To quote:

"It must be concluded that HRT-users run a smaller risk of relapse [new tumour] and mortality from breast cancer and that HRT thus does not appear to exert detrimental effects."

To offer you a numerical impression: in the HRT (estrogen) treated group the breast cancer relapse was 17 in thousand and in the control group it was 30 in thousand.[30]

In the HRT users breast mortality was 5 per 1000 and in the control group (no estrogen) it was 15 per 1000, three hundred percent higher.

It is important for the breast cancer survivor to learn on what (flimsy) grounds this BAN (use of ERT in breast cancer survivors) is based.

The main **arguments** are the following:

1) Breast cancer is clearly a hormone-dependent disease. More specifically, it is dependent on estrogen. Seventy percent of breast cancers are ER-positive, that is the cancer cell possesses 'antennae' (called 'receptors') that make the cell sensitive to estrogen. (Explanation: estrogen binds to a receptor, which, 'activated', sends signals (instructions) to the DNA in the cell nucleus).
As this may sound scary it should be pointed out that normal breast cells also possess these estrogen receptors, as do certain white blood cells.
For that reason estrogens can stimulate the growth of these tumours, so the reasoning goes.
Males also get breast cancer, but their risk is a hundred times smaller. The difference is a matter of hormones: estrogen.

2) Women with an early menarche (1st menstruation) and late menopause and so have been longer exposed to estrogens, have an increased risk of breast cancer. So the longer a woman is exposed to estrogens, the greater the risk.

3) In ER-positive breast cancers anti-estrogen medicines like tamoxifen (Nolvadex) and anastrozol (Arimidex) are effec-

---

[30] Expressed in women – years: a statistical concept.

tive in metastasized breast cancer and as supplementary therapy in primary breast cancer. So, the less the breast cancer cell is exposed to estrogen the better. Conversely, adding estrogen is perhaps throwing fuel on the fire if mini-cancers are present in the breast.

On the grounds of these arguments most oncologists (cancer specialists) and gynaecologists believe that estrogen therapy is absolutely forbidden (contra-indicated) in women who have had breast cancer in the past.

Comment: you may submit arguments 'for or against' as long as you want, statistics has the final word.
Randomized studies of breast cancer survivors provide the definitive answer.
Ex-breast cancer women (volunteers are divided in two groups by drawing lots: one gets an estrogen (ET) over a long period, the other a sugar pill (placebo)).

If it should turn out that estrogen therapy (ET) increases the risk, then the thesis 'estrogen is contra-indicated' is justified. If, however, the result would show that estrogen has no influence on the risk of new breast cancer, or even lowers the risk, then the (older) woman can safely receive estrogen therapy (ET), with all the advantages for her health and quality of life attached to it.

Conclusion:
Arguments are fine; but statistical tests provide the final answer (see below).

Contra-arguments. As I will show the arguments supplied are weak and of little consequence. This is not surprising since – as I will divulge at this early stage - statistical studies show that with the right hormone therapy estrogen does not increase the risk of recurrence.

1) It is true that 70 percent of breast cancers have 'antennae' for estrogen (ER-positive). Estrogen promotes the growth of these tumours. So, no estrogen. "True or not true?"

Estrogen antennae. Sounds ominous. But, as stated, healthy breast cells also have estrogen receptors, just like some other cell types in the body, mainly certain immune cells like (*don't be put off by unfamiliar names*) lymphocytes, macrophages, natural killer cells and dendritic cells.

The conclusion: "ER-positive means the more estrogen the faster cancer grows" is incorrect.

In this respect you can compare cancer with a sponge in a bathtub. When you remove all the water from the tub the sponge dries out. It shrinks (of course). You only have to add just a little bit of water and the sponge 'grows' by sucking up water.

But if you continue filling the bathtub the sponge is not going to grow further (full is full). That's the same with the ER-positive cancer cell.

Just as in the case of prostate cancer and testosterone the breast cancer cell needs only a minimal concentration of estrogen to grow a bit faster than without estrogen. More estrogen than this minimum does not mean faster growth of the tumour.

But when you keep the cancer cell completely 'estrogen-free' as with anti-estrogen treatment (tamoxifen) the cancer will shrink. The reverse is not true: adding more than the minimal estrogen level will not make the tumour grow faster.

Conclusion: the statement "estrogen is fuel on the fire of cancer growth" is a fallacy. This is in agreement with medical practice: in younger women who have had breast cancer the ovaries are not removed as a precaution against latent tumours or mini-tumours growing faster because of ample estrogen produced by the ovaries!

To deny the older women estrogen therapy categorically is thus to apply double standards. It doesn't make sense.

2) The role of early menarche and late menopause in the risk of breast cancer is of little import. As we saw in chapter 19 the risk is just a bit more than that of alcohol or pregnancy at an advanced age. That estrogen cannot be a big player in the causation of breast cancer already follows from the fact that breast cancer in women between 50-59 occurs 700 percent more often than in women between 30 and 39 who produce estrogens in abundance (see chapter 19).

The argument that men have a far lower risk of breast cancer carries little meaning since we know that the difference between male and female is not only a matter of hormones as previously thought, but is mainly determined by the Y-chromosome in the male and the 'extra' X-chromosome in the female (see chapter 19).

With this all three arguments against the use of estrogen presented above have been refuted.

Yet, there are a number of important scientifically based arguments to offer estrogen therapy to this group of women after a suitable 'waiting period' of, say, two to three years.

I'll just mention two in order not to burden the reader unduly. Of course it concerns women in (after) the menopause.

1) Estrogen causes – don't be put off by the term – apoptosis ('suicide' by the cell) in breast cancer cells.

Incidentally, this is historically of interest for it explains why doctors prior to 1970 treated ER-positive breast tumours in older women with high doses of estrogens to induce tumour regression. The success rate was about 50 percent.[31]

After the development of tamoxifen this approach was abandoned. This favourable action of estrogen on breast cancer cells (apoptosis) is the more effective the longer the cancer has been exposed

---

[31] Estrogen regulation of apoptosis: how can one hormone stimulate and inhibit? J.S. Lewis and V.C. Jordan: Breast Cancer Research, 11, 206, 2009.

to an estrogen-poor environment. So it is e.g. more effective in eliminating remaining cancer cells 5 years after the cessation of menstruation than shortly after.

Conclusion: in menopausal women estrogen can contribute to eliminating latent or remaining cancer cells by stimulating the cell mechanism called apoptosis (suicide).

The main mechanism whereby estrogen contributes to eliminating remaining or potential cancer cells is however the immune system.

This topic deserves our special attention, so it deserves a special heading.

Estrogens and cancer defence
If you have survived cancer, but also if you never had cancer your chances of remaining cancer-free are better when your immune system is in optimal shape.

Let's not forget in this connection that one in three persons will get cancer.

Take your time to 'study' this section, which has a direct bearing on the question "to use or not to use estrogen after breast cancer".

Just as our immune system continually attacks and destroys bacteria to prevent sepsis ('blood poisoning'), so newly formed malignant cells are constantly identified, attacked and destroyed by this defence mechanism.

The weaker the immune system, the greater the risk of cancer.

The classical example is AIDS, in which the so-called T-lymphocytes of the immune system are decimated by the HIV virus. Result: young people get malignant tumours, among which the notorious Kaposi sarcoma, which is even the first symptom in thirty percent of cases.

Still more telling is the fact that organ transplantation patients who have to use immune-suppressive drugs to prevent organ rejection have a 100-300 times higher risk of cancer. Mind you, not 300 percent, but 300 times, almost mind-boggling!

This single fact alone proves the huge significance of the immune system for our defence against cancer.

Lesson: the stronger the immune system the better you're protected against cancer.

There is even a special term for this defence against pre-cancerous cells and cancer cells: **cancer immunological surveillance.**

This concept was introduced in 1957 by the world-famous Nobel Prize winner professor MacFarlene Burnet to represent the fact that lymphocytes act as guards that continuously identify early malignant cells and destroy them.

In the frame below further information is provided.

> **Immunological surveillance** is of extreme importance for the elimination of malignant and pre-malignant cells and induces the death of abnormal cells by the direct action of IFN-gamma (apoptosis) and – indirectly - by stimulating the production of chemokines, that - besides other actions - block angioneogenesis (formation of new blood vessels) and thereby starve the developing tumour. Natural Killer cells, macrophages and tumour specific CDR+T-cells complete the slaughter in the final stages of the immune response.

Just like the armed forces consist of different units (infantry, engineering corps, intelligence service, etc.) so the immune system consists of sub-divisions which each have their own task. I'll just mention: - don't get put off by unfamiliar terms - Natural Killer cells, lymphocytes, macrophages and dendritic cells.

Why do I mention these different cell types? Because they are all involved in the fight against cancer and are ER-positive, that is, that they, just like healthy breast cells and most breast cancer cells, possess estrogen 'antennae' (estrogen receptors).

This is by the way also the case in the male in whom estradiol is locally made from testosterone by the enzyme aromatase.

This estrogen dependence of the immune system perhaps explains why women have a somewhat stronger immune system than men and live on the average five years longer.

The exquisite sensitivity of the immune system to the estrogen level is well illustrated by the fact that the number of Natural Killer cells (short-lived lymphocytes that kill cancer cells) is two times higher before ovulation, when the estradiol level is at its highest, than during the second half of the cycle.

This is not too surprising since nature never does anything without a reason: the estradiol receptors (antennae) on the white blood cells have a function: **activation**.

To offer an example: estradiol, through its action via the receptors, activates a number of genes in macrophages (a type of white blood cells), which enables them to destroy cancer cells more effectively.[32]

To end this section I'll just mention that - as may be expected – the immune system is still active in the presence of an existing cancer, but just like in the battle between the police and the Mafia the immune system may fail.

Incidentally, in breast tumours where the tumour is infiltrated by lymphocytes (so-called CD+8 lymphocytes) the prognosis is much more favourable than in tumours without infiltration (weak immune system.[33]

With this I would like to end the discussion of 'background arguments'.

It should be clear that the arguments to categorically prohibit the use of estrogens after breast cancer are in flat contradiction to the latest scientific findings and views. On the contrary, the scientific findings 'predict' that estrogen therapy after 'cured' breast cancer in 50+ women offers protection against new breast cancers, or is at least neutral, that is, does not increase the risk of recurrence.

Who has the last word, the final say, the decisive voice? The statistician, that is, statistical research in which two groups are compared: breast cancer 'survivors' receiving ET (estrogen therapy) and those who don't (control group).

---

32 Kramer, P.R., Estradiol regulates expression of genes that function in macrophage activation. Journal of Steroid Biochemistry and Molecular Biology, 279, no.3, 203, 2002.
33 For example, Aaltomaa et.al. state, "lymphocytes infiltrates were related to a good outcome in breast cancer, especially in rapidly proliferating tumours". See Aaltomaa, S. et al. Lymphocyte infiltrates as a prognostic variable in female breast cancer. Eur. J. Cancer, 28A, 859, 1992.

Statistical studies: the deciding vote
Because statistics is not common fare I'll start by pointing out that the golden standard is 'randomized' study. This means that the subjects are assigned by lot in two groups. One group gets the 'drug' (here estrogen) while the other receives a sugar pill (placebo).

Thus far (2013) only two 'randomized' studies have been carried out and they will be discussed at the end of this section.

Let me begin by presenting the result of a so-called *meta-analysis*, whereby the results of all published studies are treated as a single whole and statistically analysed (by the way: statistics is a branch of applied mathematics, a difficult field of study).

In a 2006 paper entitled, "Menopausal hormone therapy (HT) in patients with breast cancer" the researchers study (quote): 'the action of estrogen therapy on the recurrence, cancer-related mortality and total mortality after breast cancer diagnosis.' [So, it concerns breast cancer survivors.]

All available studies were 'thrown together' and analysed as a whole.

I am not going to tire you with numbers, but only mention the final results.

In the conclusion the researchers state: "…. HT use in breast cancer survivors was not associated with increased cancer recurrence, cancer-related mortality or total mortality." On the contrary. The report says, "Compared to non-users HT patients had a lower risk of breast cancer recurrence and cancer-related mortality."

In other words, analysis of all published studies shows that – in glaring contrast to the view of most oncologists and gynaecologists – that there is not a shred of evidence that estrogen therapy (ET) after breast cancer constitutes a risk.

In order not to burden the poor reader unduly the list of studies and their conclusions is put in a frame.

Statistical observational studies in random order.

J Natl Cancer Inst.93, 764, 2001
Hormone replacement therapy after a diagnosis of breast cancer in relation to recurrence and mortality.
O'Meary et.al.

Conclusion: We found a lower risk for cancer recurrence and mortality. The results show that HRT after breast cancer has no adverse influence on recurrence and mortality.

Climacteric.7, 384, 2004
Hormone replacement therapy after a diagnosis of breast cancer: cancer recurrence.
Durna EM et.al.

Conclusion: HRT is not associated with an increased risk of cancer recurrence or shortened life expectancy.

Maturitas, 53, 123, 2006
Menopausal hormone therapy (HT) in patients with breast cancer.
Batur, P. et. al.

Conclusion: In our study HT use after menopause in breast cancer survivors was not associated with an increased cancer recurrence, cancer mortality or total mortality.

Int. J. Fert. Womens Med, 44, 186, 1999
An experience with estrogen replacement therapy in breast cancer survivors.
Brerster, W.R., et.al.

Conclusion: The concern that ERT could activate the growth of occult metastases and could promote an explosion of new tumours was not corroborated.

Ann Surg Oncol, 8, 828, 2001
Estrogen therapy after breast cancer: a 12-year follow-up.
Peters G.N., et. al.

Conclusion: The use of ERT in a group of breast cancer survivors with tumours with a good prognosis was not associated with increased cancer risks.

Menopause, 10, 277, 2003
Estrogen replacement therapy in breast cancer survivors: a matched-controlled study.
Decker, D.A. .et.al.

Conclusion: ERT did not result in new cancers or metastases.

Med J Aust,7, 177, 2002
Hormone replacement therapy after a diagnosis of breast cancer, cancer recurrence and mortality.
Durna E.M., et. al.

Conclusion: HRT use in women treated for invasive breast cancer is not associated with an increased risk of breast cancer recurrence or shortened life expectancy.

J Fam Pract, 51, 1056, 2002
Cancer recurrence in women using hormone replacement therapy: meta-analysis.
Maurer, L.H., Lens, S.

Conclusion: Current research does not support the universal withholding of ERT to well-informed women with low-grade breast cancer.

Am J Clin. Oncol., 23, 64, 2000
Breast cancer survival and hormone replacement therapy: a cohort analysis.
Disala, O.J.et .al.

Conclusion: This analysis shows that HRT after the treatment of breast cancer is not associated with adverse effects.

Gynaecol Obsstet Fert, 32, 614.2003
Hormonereplacement therapy in breast cancer patients: a study of 230 patients, with a case-control study.
Gorins,A. et .al.

Conclusion: the quality of life was often greatly improved and a harmful effect on the cancer disease was not found.

Oncology 60, 199, 2001
Hormone replacement therapy after treatment of breast cancer: effects on postmenopausal symptoms, bone mineral and recurrence rates.
Beckmann,M.W.et .al.

Conclusion: There were no statistical differences with regard to course of the disease and mortality [So, no adverse effects, JGD]

J Clin Oncol, 17, 1482, 1999
Estrogen replacement therapy after localized breast cancer: clinical outcome of 319 women followed prospectively.
Selli , R., et .al.

Conclusion: ERT does not increase the risk of breast cancer recurrence, nor does it influence the course of the disease.

Am J Obstet Gynaecol, 174, 1494, 1996
Hormone replacement therapy in breast cancer survivors: a cohort study.
Disala. P.J. et .al.

Conclusion: No adverse effect could be found in this study.

Am J Obstet Gynaecol, 181, 288, 1999
Estrogen replacement therapy in women with previous breast cancer.
Natrajan P.K. et.al.

Conclusion: ERT does not increase cancer recurrence or mortality.

Am J Obstet Gynaecol, 187 289, 2002
Estrogen replacement therapy in patients with early breast cancer.
Natrajan, P.K. and Gambrell, R.D. Jr.

Conclusion: ERT does not increase the risk of recurrence or mortality in patients with early [cured] breast cancer.

Int J Gynaecol Obstet, 64, 59, 1999
Estrogen replacement therapy in breast cancer survivors.
Guidozzi, F.

Conclusion: Breast cancer survivors did not have their outcome adversely affected by ERT during an observation period of 22-44 months.

J Nat Cancer Inst, 93, 754, 2001
Hormone replacement therapy after a diagnosis of breast cancer in relation to the recurrence and mortality.
O'Meary, E.S. et .al.

Conclusion: We found a lower risk for recurrence and mortality in women who used ERT after the cancer diagnosis than in women who did not. The results show that HRT has no adverse effect on recurrence and mortality.

> **Final note**
> The fact that doctors are often put on the wrong track is not surprising because of the complex actions of estrogen. Estrogens can stimulate the growth of cancer cells in tissue culture in low doses, but on the contrary inhibit the growth in high doses.
> Breast cancers are able to regulate and maintain their internal levels of estradiol independent of the concentration outside the tumour, so the estrogen replacement has little or no influence on tumour growth (see Blankenstein, M.A. et.al., J Steroid Biochem Mol Biol 41, 891, 1993).

The crucial role of natural estrogens (estradiol, estriol, etc.) on strengthening the immune system is often totally ignored in theoretical discussions and considerations.

We will now reach the dénouement? How's that?

Because only randomised studies (assigned by lot) can offer the definitive answer.

Thus far (2014) two important randomised studies have been carried out, both in Sweden. The result?

In 1997 two randomised studies were started in Sweden. Let me start with a discussion of the study called **HABITS** (acronym for: hormonal replacement therapy after breast cancer – is it safe?)

As I explained earlier, in randomised studies the test persons (here breast cancer survivors) are assigned by lot in two groups: the treated group and the control group.

After three years the **HABITS**-study was prematurely terminated because women in the HT group had more new cancer complications than those in the control group.

The results were published in 2004 (Lancet, 363, 453, 2004) and in 2008 (J Natl Cancer Inst 100, 475, 2008).

A surprising and disappointing result!

However, what was the case? Just as in the WHI study (chapter19) whereby women on Prempro (combination preparation of estrogen and a progestin) had a higher cancer risk due to the added progestin, this was also the case here. Not the estrogen but the added progestin (artificial variant of progesterone) was the culprit.

That this progestin was the cause was proven by the result of a second Swedish study, the so-called **Stockholm study.**

As the researchers write the main purpose of the Stockholm study was (quote), "to minimize the use of progestin (progestogen)."

The result after 4 years was that (quote), "**the risk of breast cancer recurrence was unrelated to HRT [estrogen therapy].**"

In a 2012 paper (Eur. J Cancer, Aug., 2012) the investigators of the Stockholm study state, "After a follow-up period of 10.8 years there was no difference in breast cancer events between the HRT group and the control group." Furthermore they conclude, "The increased breast cancer recurrence in HABITS is due to too high exposure to progestin."

Conclusion: the randomized Stockholm study shows that breast cancer survivors treated with estrogen only (with minimal addition of progestin) have no increased risk for the recurrence of breast cancer and other complications.

Although the Stockholm study too is not perfect, since it had to be terminated prematurely because of the false alarm raised by the HABITS study, we may, taking all statistical studies into consideration (both 'observational' and 'randomized'), conclude that properly applied ERT (e.g. estradiol and only four times a year progesterone added) poses no risk whatsoever with regard to breast cancer recurrence and other cancer complications.

The taboo ('contra-indication') regarding estrogen therapy in breast cancer survivors is wrong and totally unjustified.

Afterword
Since ERT has no adverse effect on breast tissue and on the prognosis in breast cancer survivors the well-informed 50+ woman should seriously consider estrogen replacement therapy in order to prevent conditions and diseases caused by estrogen deficiency (see chapter 19), including osteoporosis, premature heart problems, stroke and increased risk of dying. For many women the prospect of 'feminine forever' has its own sex-appeal.

Be in charge
The health-conscious, well-informed individual should make his/her own decisions in matters such as these.

Just like it is up to the woman and not the doctor to use (or not to use) 'the Pill', so, for the 50+ woman the choice to use ERT (estrogen) should be hers, not the doctor's. But since most doctors are ill-informed about this subject, it may not be easy to get his/her cooperation. If your physician is not an authoritarian figure you might invite him to read chapter 19 (and 19A) of this book.

But the intelligent, determined woman – exemplified by Suzanne Somers, American celebrity - will always find a way and a doctor to obtain this life-preserving hormone: estradiol. Good hunting ...

Chapter 20

Testosteron, the hormone of life

While in the female the production of the sex hormone stops abruptly after 50, the sex hormone production in the male gradually decreases, so that after 60 the value of the available testosterone (the so-called free testosterone) is only less than a third of an 18-year-old, falling to minimal values after 80.

A normal phenomenon, which however constitutes a threat to life expectancy, increases the risk of cardiovascular diseases and lowers the quality of life. *Old-age: so, 'normal'*. But just as the older man gets reading glasses and implants for his lost teeth, so the older man should receive testosterone supplementation for maintaining quality of life and extending his lifespan.

This is not a choice that the doctor should make but (using a fancy term) an 'existential choice' the older 'life-extender' should make for himself.

But let me start with a curious anomalous finding.
If you want to live a very long life you should have yourself castrated at an early age in your next incarnation. Eunuchs live quite a bit longer. Korean scientists studied the birth and deaths registries of Korea's Chosun Dynasty from 1302-1910 and were able to show that eunuchs on the average live 16 years longer than normal.[34]

Conclusion:
So, the lower the testosterone level the better? Wrong. What holds for eunuchs does not hold for men with a low testosterone level.

On the contrary: the lower the testosterone level the higher the risk of dying from all causes, but especially from cardiac condi-

---
[34] Kyung-Jin Min e.a., Current Biology, 22, R792, 2012.

tions. This is the outcome of a Cambridge study involving 12,000 men over a period of 4 years (1993-1997). After excluding other factors it was found that men with the lowest testosterone values (so-called lowest quartile) had a forty percent higher risk of dying in the next ten years than men with the highest testosterone values (highest quartile).[35]

There are numerous studies that show the relationship between low testosterone values and the increased risk of dying. A 18-year study of older men under the telling title "Low Serum Testosterone and Mortality in Older Men"[36] showed that the 30 percent with the lowest testosterone values had a 33 percent higher risk of dying within the next 18 years than men with higher testosterone. The lesson? Make sure that your testosterone level is maintained, unless you are tired of living, which by the way may well be a sign of too little testosterone.

But as a 60+ male do you have to have a much too low testosterone – lower than 300ng/dl - to qualify for testosterone replacement?

Yes, according to your doctor. No, according to biological logic and the needs of your organism.

As mentioned, men over 60 have less than one-third of the available testosterone (so-called free testosterone) of their youth. Even if there are no symptoms this is - from the biological viewpoint - not a desirable state of affairs. For both men and women the iron rule holds: "Decreased sex hormone production due to aging accelerates the aging process and risk of dying." So, a vicious circle.

Decreased testosterone → increased aging → decreased testosterone → increased aging, etc.

As a result: increased risk of aging diseases, including cardiovascular diseases, Alzheimer and cancer.

Just a remark before proceeding. The older 'life-extender' should always be able to find a doctor to prescribe testosterone supple-

---
35 Kay-Tee Kwaw e.a., Circulation, 116, 2094, 2007.
36 Laughlin, G.A. e.a. Journal of Clinical Endocrinology and Metabolism, 93, 68, 2007.

mentation, even when there are no symptoms and his testosterone tests are 'normal' for his age. As a ploy of last resort you could even claim impotence, or present this chapter to your doctor. If you're bold and 60+ try to find an internist in the hospital with the request for testosterone replacement therapy to prevent osteoporosis or find a complementary doctor who is often more open to orthomolecular medicine that includes hormone replacement.

In order to give you a clear idea how 'testosterone-deficit' increases with age let me mention de following figures. In men between 20-40 years 2 percent has a (too) low bio-available testosterone (this is the fraction not bound to protein).
In men between 40-49 this percentage is 7 percent.
Between 50-59 this value is 30 percent, between 60-69 43 percent and between 70-79 over 70 percent.

What does this mean? A too low testosterone level is called hypogonadism in younger men: underactive gonads (testis). This is similar to hypothyroidism, a syndrome caused by an underactive thyroid gland. The symptoms of hypogonadism are among others lack of libido, erectile dysfunction, easy fatigue, poor sleep, high cholesterol, depression, anxiety, mental dullness, lack of initiative and joie de vivre, diminished quality of life and a tendency towards obesity and breast formation.

In the 50+ male these are 'normal' symptoms of aging. Normal, my foot! If you're over fifty and you recognize this picture as applying to you, you're in the andropause, the equivalent of the menopause.
There is a simple solution: replacement with testosterone.

If you are 60+ and are symptom–free, fit and healthy, it is advisable from the perspective of anti-aging, 'life-extension', and prevention (cardiac problems, Alzheimer, diabetes, osteoporosis, etc.) to use testosterone supplementation (replacement). That with this the quality of life is often improved is of course a welcome 'side-effect'.
But before proceeding with the practical aspects an important

question needs to be addressed: "Does testosterone replacement activate the growth of prostate cancer or 'latent' prostate cancer?"
This is the subject of the next section.

Testosterone and prostate cancer: the myth
Since time immemorial the myth prevails among doctors in general and urologists in particular that testosterone a) activates 'dormant' prostate cancers and b) makes prostate cancer grow faster (fuel to the fire).

Just like the myth in cardiology, "Three eggs a week at the most" and the myth in gynaecology, "Estrogen activates breast cancer" (see chapter 19A) the myth "Testosterone supplementation activates prostate cancer, both dormant an active" is accepted as a truism in urology and beyond.

In 2006 this myth was exposed as a myth by the Harvard urologist professor A. Morgentaler in a paper with the telling title "Testosterone and prostate cancer: A historical perspective on a modern myth." which appeared in 2006 (European Urology, 50, 935, 2006).[37]

The myth is partially based on the observation that in cases of prostate cancer castration or estrogen therapy (both eliminate testosterone production) causes the tumour to shrink. So, no testosterone, a smaller tumour.

Adding testosterone to a castrate with prostate cancer results in tumour growth.
Conclusion: testosterone is like fuel to the fire in prostate cancer. Professor Morgentaler and others have shown in a series of studies that this 'extrapolation' (conclusion) is wrong.

Beyond a very low level of testosterone the tumour does not grow any faster. It is, what is called, a threshold phenomenon.

The situation is like in a sponge in a bathtub.

---

37 See also Morgentaler, A., Testosterone Replacement Therapy and Prostate Cancer, Urol Clin N Am 14, 555, 2007.

If you empty the bathtub the sponge will shrink (no water). If you fill the bath again the sponge 'grows' by sucking up water until it is 'full'.

After that it grows no further however much water is added to the tub. So the myth is partly based on a 'funny thought' (wrong extrapolation) which seems obvious but is wrong.

A second – far more shocking – aspect of this myth is that the 'clinical evidence' that was presented by the urologist Dr. Higgins in 1941 consisted of three patients of whom only one served the purpose. Dr. Morgentaler - myth-breaker and Sherlock Holmes - discovered this long-forgotten paper in the Harvard library gathering dust. He writes, "Dr. Higgins had based his 'accelerated growth' conclusion on one single patient, using a blood test – acid phosphatase - that has long since been abandoned because of its unreliability."

Dr. Morgentaler was flabbergasted, couldn't believe his eyes (he wrote in his book): A 70-year-old myth (a truism for all doctors) based on the evidence of a single patient and a 'nutty thought'. But a medical myth, however false, is very persistent, like the cardiologist's myth, 'No more than three eggs a week'.

In his book *Testosterone for Life* Dr. Morgentaler concludes, "Dr. Higgins' assertion that higher testosterone caused greater growth of prostate cancer, repeated for so long and accepted as gospel, was based on almost nothing at all."

That the assertion "The higher the testosterone level the greater the risk of prostate cancer" is wrong even the layman can gather from the fact that prostate cancer rarely occurs at an early age when the testosterone level is highest, but mainly at a later age when the testosterone level is low or very low.

I would like to end this section with the observation that in a large number of studies involving a total of 430,000 men in none of them an association was found between testosterone levels and prostate cancer. The largest and best executed study (so-called 'prospective' study) even found an inverse relation between the risk of prostate cancer and testosterone level, that is, the higher the T-level the lower the risk.

Conclusion:
Professor Morgentaler concludes:
Testosterone replacement has no adverse effect on prostate cancer risk, does not activate 'dormant' micro-prostate cancers, and does not increase the growth of prostate cancer.

Testosterone after 50+
Not for your libido, sex or muscle power, but for slowing down the aging process (vicious circle, see above), for a drastic reduction of the risk of dying and the risk of cardio-vascular diseases, osteoporosis, Alzheimer, kidney failure, etc. it is advisable to keep your testosterone after 50 at a youthful level.

For the female this is simple. After the start of the menopause the value of the main sex hormone, estradiol, is less than 10 percent of its youthful value. So, for the female life-extender the choice is straightforward: ERT.

For the male, especially between 50 and 60, the situation is less black and white, but as a rule of thumb we may assume that from age 35 on the testosterone level decreases by 1 percent a year, that is 10 percent per decade. So, at 55 (rule of thumb) your testosterone level is 20 percent lower than when you were young and 30 percent lower at 65.

Since there is, even at younger ages, a large spread in normal testosterone values (between 400 and 1000 ng/dl) it is not necessary – like in thyroid hormone supplementation – to stay within a small range. Although it certainly makes sense to measure the blood testosterone level, such a measurement has limited significance. Why? In the first place because the common test, the measurement of (so-called) total testosterone (TT), does not present a reliable picture of the bio-available testosterone, the (so-called) free testosterone, that is, the testosterone not bound to protein. The free testosterone is only about 2 percent of the total testosterone and most clinical methods to determine the free testosterone leave much to be desired.

The interested reader can find the technical details in the frame below

> Testosterone circulates in the bloodstream in three forms: the free testosterone (unbound), testosterone bound to albumin and testosterone bound to SHBG (sex hormone binding globulin).
> The free testosterone is directly biologically available (so, active), the albumin bound testosterone is 'potentially' available because of its loose binding to the protein albumin, while the testosterone that is tightly bound to SHBG (also a protein) is biologically inactive.
> As mentioned, commonly only the total testosterone (TT) is determined. Since the SHBG concentration rises with age, resulting in a higher percentage of the total testosterone being bound to SHBG, the determination of TT in the older individual is often misleading or meaningless.
> The TT-value may be normal (400ng/dl, say) while there is still a testosterone deficit because a higher percentage is bound to SHBG.
> Only when the TT-value is too low (300ng/dl or lower) the result is unambiguous: there is definitely a deficit.
> So, the best test is the measurement of free testosterone. A number of methods are in use, but the method recommended by the leading expert in this field, professor Morgentaler, is the so-called analogue free testosterone test, also known as the RIA test. In most clinical labs this test is used.
> A value below 15 pg/ml) determined by the RIA method definitely indicates a deficit, even in the absence of any symptoms.
> In most cases the testosterone test is superfluous in men over 60, as their testosterone production is considerably less than in their best years.

Practical aspects of testosterone replacement
If you contemplate addition to the family you shouldn't use testosterone supplementation as it may lower your sperm count.

A potential risk of TR (testosterone replacement) in younger men is that it may (by its action on the hypothalamus) lower the body's own production of the hormone. For men over 60 this is not a problem as the supplementation greatly overshadows the small decrease of testosterone production in the testicles.

Testosterone preparations
Currently (2014) the following preparations are available:
  A gel, applied to the upper arm: Testim and Androgel
  Oral: Andriol (2-4 capsules a day)
  Long-acting (intramuscular) injection (3 months) Nebido
  This requires the help of your doctor.

I wish you good luck in trying to persuade your doctor to write a prescription. Otherwise find another one: your very life may be at stake (see 'statistics' above).

Chapter 21

The birth control pill is very harmful

The Pill acts by largely switching off the function of the ovaries. This implies that the production of (natural) estrogens drops to slightly above the level in the menopause. The blood level of the most important estrogen, estradiol, has, in the fertile period, a mean value of 250 pg/ml.[38]

The estradiol blood level of the woman on the pill is on the average 25 pg/ml, so, only one-tenth of the normal mean value.

The estradiol value in the menopause is a bit lower than 10 pg/ml.

Thus, the woman on the Pill is hormonally a virtual 'castrate' and is in a condition comparable to the menopause.

The consequences of a deficit of natural estrogens (estradiol) are discussed in depth in chapter 19. The reader is invited to (re)read chapter 19 carefully before proceeding. Estrogen deficit accelerates the aging process and much more, with all its future consequences.

This has also been shown at the level of the cell: it was shown in older women that the shorter they had been exposed to their own estrogen production (late menarche, early menopause) the shorter the telomeres (see chapter 13), the time clock of aging at the level of the cell, the building block of our body.[39]

The length of the telomeres determines the biological age of the individual. In a group of people of the same age, those with short telomeres are biologically older than individuals with longer telomeres.

The woman who uses the Pill for many years is only exposed for a brief period to her own (normal) estrogen production. The shorten-

---

38 The value fluctuates strongly during the menstrual cycle and individual values vary widely.
39 Blackburn, E., et.al., Greater endogenous estrogen exposure is associated with longer telomeres, Brain Res., 1379, 224, 2011.

ing of the telomeres is comparable to women who enter the menopause before the age of 40, as is the case in 3 percent of women.

'But the Pill does contain estrogen, doesn't it?' the reader may object. 'Isn't that sufficient to compensate for the loss of the body's own production?'

Yes, the Pill does contain estrogen, actually a synthetic (artificial) estrogen, usually (don't be put off by a name) ethinylestradiol.

Why do most birth control pills contain this substance? To compensate for the loss of estrogens produced by the ovaries? No, because this synthetic substance shuts off the function of the ovaries (via suppressing the pituitary gland), thus preventing pregnancy.

Initially, in the sixties, the dosage was 'high': 50 microgram. As ethinylestradiol was shown to cause thrombosis (death) and stroke, the dosage has been considerably lowered to values below 30 microgram, or even zero. In the latter case the Pill only contains a progestin, an artificial variant of the natural hormone progesterone.

This low 'safe' dose of ethinylestradiol hardly offers any compensation for the loss of your own estrogen production. The woman on the current Pill is like a woman in the menopause who is treated with a totally inadequate HT (hormone therapy), both in terms of dose and choice of hormone. This synthetic estrogen exerts very different biological actions on the body as the natural hormone estradiol. One example suffices to illustrate the point: estradiol does not cause thrombosis, ethinylestradiol does.

In 1997 an editorial appeared in the Dutch Journal of Medicine written by professor James Defares entitled **The influence of birth control pills on the woman.**
The summary is presented below.

Summary
Many recent studies have led to the conclusion that long-term use of birth control pills lead to the suppression of the endogenous [own] estrogen production, while no study shows that the estrogen component in the pill can be considered sufficient compensation for the decreased production.
This leads to the conclusion that long-term use of the pill leads to chronic estrogen deficiency and thus to damage to all somatic and mental functions of the organism, while it promotes the development of osteoporosis and atherosclerosis.
In the light of all recent studies the conclusion seems justified that the use of the present pill by women in the fertile period leads to acceleration of the process of aging.

This was long ago, but since then the situation hasn't changed; on the contrary, it has only grown worse since the estrogen content in the current birth control pills is only half (or less) than in the sixties: 30 microgram or zero instead of 50 microgram.

So, to repeat: the woman on the pill is in the condition of the woman in the menopause who is treated with a harmful artificial hormone (ethinylestradiol) in a dose which is far too low to compensate for the virtual loss of her own estrogen production.

Is that all? No, it is far worse.

Most birth control pills contain two components 1) a synthetic estrogen and 2) a progestin, a synthetic variant of the pregnancy hormone progesterone.

There are dozens of different kinds of progestin, some more harmful than others. Just one example: some progestins possess testosterone – like properties that not only result in defeminisation (due to lack of estrogen) but to masculinization, including undesirable hair, voice changes, and even sometimes lesbian feelings.

Below I'll just present a random sample from the mire of the taking of the Pill.

Loss of libido, depression, abnormal fatigue, hypertension (the Pill is the main cause of high blood pressure in young women), dulling of emotional life (both the 'emotional centre' and the 'sex centre' are located in the hypothalamus, that part of the brain targeted by the Pill), are common.

The symptoms and degenerative effects are the result of the combined action of serious estrogen deficit and the toxic influence of the progestin. Researchers have found (also in identical twins) that women on the Pill are judged less attractive and less feminine by men than women without the Pill.

The Pill disturbs the glucose-insulin metabolism in the sense that the pancreas must produce far more insulin (up to 5 times more) than normal to keep the glucose level in check, something that is clinically unnoticed because the glucose values are normal. The milder side-effects include hair loss, weight gain by water retention, melasma - fanciful 'birthmarks' on the face – and 'ectropion', a cauliflower-like benign tumour at the neck of the womb. I have observed this a number of times in my practice and when I showed it to the woman via a mirror or a picture she would almost pass out. Gynaecologists (in the Netherlands) would shrug their shoulders and call it soothingly (in the sixties) a Lyndiol–cauliflower. A drug that produces such horrible deformities does not belong in a healthy body. It may be mentioned in passing that the Pill, as you may read in Wikipedia, increases breast cancer risk by 24 percent, virtually the same percentage that was found in the harmful combination pill for the menopause, Prempro, that caused such commotion world-wide. (See chapter 19 for a full discussion).

It would take a whole book to discuss all harmful and undesirable effects of the Pill, such as my 1970 book Autumn in Spring (out of print). The interested reader is advised to read the well-known book of the medical reporter Barbara Seaman *The Doctor's Case Against the Pill* (latest edition 1995). This book - a litany of medical misery - prompted the Gaylord Nelson's Senate Hearings over Pill Safety – a landmark event.

The woman who after reading this chapter in connection with chapter 19 still considers using the Pill or staying on the Pill is (excuse me) a self-destructing fool.

"But what is the alternative?" you would wonder in despair. Back to the detested condom?

For most women the IUD is the best solution.
But beware of signs of infection, a condition when neglected becomes chronic and may lead to infertility.

Chapter 22

The fundamental cause of aging: the telomere

Aging and death (lifespan) are closely related. Everybody knows it: the faster you age the shorter your life expectancy and conversely.

Why do we age, why do we die after 60?
Simply because nature is only interested in the survival of the species, not in the fate of the individual.
The woman bears children between 20 and 40. The children have to be protected by their parents until adulthood. So the parents have to stay fit and healthy till 60.
Nature couldn't care less about what happens after 60. The continuity of the species is assured.
You could compare it with a cheap watch. The guarantee is 2 years. What happens after that is of no concern to the producer. But the watch will not self-destruct after the guarantee period. That would be too expensive. But it is allowed to decay.
Or the space probe Voyager 2 developed to take pictures of Jupiter and Neptune. NASA developed the space probe so it would function perfectly for 5 years. The probe continues its voyage into infinity.
But what happens to the probe beyond Neptune NASA couldn't care less, although it is still in top condition 40 years after its launch.

Philosophically true and interesting, but it tells us nothing about the mechanism of the aging process.
Although in the past 120 years a number of speculative theories have been proposed over aging, varying from the 'wear and tear' theory from 1882 by the renowned biologist August Weismann to the DNA mutation theory, there is only one that deserves our attention in this introduction to our main theme: the **Free Radical Theory.**

'Oops, what is that again?' It is not a political doctrine but refers to the power plants in our cells, the mitochondria (plural).

When we compare the cell to a kiwi then the mitochondria are the black pits in the kiwi. Each cell has some 500 - 1000 mitochondria (singular: mitochondrion) where the energy is produced by 'burning' glucose with the aid of oxygen. Your lungs breathe oxygen. Transported by the haemoglobin in the bloodstream it arrives at the cell where it performs its real job: producing energy in the mitochondrion with CO_2 and H_2O (water) as waste products.

But just as with our electric plants harmful waste products are also released. The coal plant produces sulphur dioxide, the atomic plant radioactive substances, etc. Our energy plants, the mitochondria, produce *free radicals* as waste-products, such as the aggressive hydrogen peroxide, or H_2O_2 (a molecule consisting of 2 hydrogen en 2 oxygen atoms). I'm not going to explain the nature of free radicals (everyone knows the term, but almost nobody knows what it really entails). The only thing you should know is that free radicals are very aggressive molecules that damage other molecules (proteins, DNA, etc.) in their direct environment.

> A free radical is a molecule or atom with at least one unpaired electron, making it very aggressive because it will 'steal' an electron from another molecule to restore the normal condition of two electrons. X-rays too produce free electrons in the body, the reason why they are harmful.

What is the essence of the Free Radical Theory of aging (and death)?

The theory proposes that aging is the result of continuous damage of biomolecules (even cholesterol) and so cells and tissues by free radicals produced by the mitochondria. And like a defective coal plant produces more sulphur dioxide than a new one, so a defective mitochondrion produces more free radicals than a flawless one.

So a vicious circle develops. The free radicals damage the mitochondrion itself, by which this damaged energy plant produces more free radicals than an undamaged one. Etc.

The older the person the more free radicals it produces, as has been shown experimentally in test animals and man. Despite the fact that the cell has its own antioxidants at its disposal (enzymes like SOD, vitamins E and C, etc.), the damage to DNA, cell membranes etc. lead to aging and death.

This is the essence of the Free Radical Theory of aging, which has been the most widely accepted theory of aging in the second half of the last century.

The 21st century has swept away all previous theories by the experimental discovery of the true cause of aging: the shortening of the telomeres (see chapter 13). The only theory still standing (till 2011) is the Free Radical Theory of Aging, which is experimentally fairly well supported.

So the dilemma is, as will become clear shortly: two well-founded theories on aging (The Telomere Theory and the Free Radical Theory) and only one can be the fundamental one, so the only one. The solution is as simple as it is surprising: the shortening of the telomeres accelerates the production of free radicals in the mitochondria.

The DNA theory of aging
Initially there were a dozen theories of aging, then only two and since 2012 only one. Gerontology - the science of aging - has finally become mature. The date? November 2011: the publication date of Sahin's paper in the leading scientific journal Nature *that* changed everything.

To use an exaggerated picture: just as the discovery of the Higgs' particle at CERN confirmed the validity of the so-called Standard theory in physics, so the findings of Sahin et. al. establish the validity of the Telomere Theory as the fundamental cause of the aging process. In other words as the only game in town.

In order to save space and your patience I would urge you to read chapter 13 on telomeres once more for background information.

In a nutshell, to refresh your memory: telomeres are the end of chromosomes. (If you compare a chromosome to a shoelace, then the plastic piece at the end is the telomere.)

The telomere is the time clock of the cell. During each cell division the telomere gets a bit shorter and after some 60 cell divisions the telomere is 'finished', no more. The result? Either the cell dies or stays on as a 'poisonous', worn-out cell, the so-called senescent cell.

If the cell produces enough of the miracle enzyme telomerase the cell can continue to multiply forever (under the right conditions): the cell 'stays young' forever, like our sex cells or germ cells in the testis. The cause of aging is the shortening of the telomeres in the cell nucleus.

What did Sahin and his group find?
They have bred mice with very short, poorly functioning telomeres. In these test animals the mitochondria performed poorly, their number per cell was much lower than normal and the production of free radicals had strongly increased.

When in these mice the telomere function and length was restored by manipulating the telomerase genes, the function (and number) of the mitochondria was normalised.

Also the mechanism of the dependence of the mitochondria on the telomeres (DNA) could be unlocked (see frame).

With this it has been shown experimentally that the condition of the mitochondria is completely dependent on the telomeres, which means that the so-called DNA theory, or more specific, the Telomere Theory (of aging), is the only one left standing, *the only game in town*. To repeat: the fundamental cause of aging is the shortening of our telomeres.

In the frame the details are presented for the scientist.

Under the title, 'Telomere Dysfunction Induces Metabolic and Mitochondrial Compromise' the study offers a clear understanding of aging and aging diseases by linking telomere dysfunction to a decrease of mitochondrial function and number.

By eliminating the telomerase gene the scientists were able, after four generations, to produce mice with extremely short telomeres. The absence of telomerase (and the presence of these short telomeres) resulted in big changes in the genes regulating the mitochondrial function and antioxidant protection (defence against free radicals by enzymes such as SOD, catalase, etc.).

What is the molecular mechanism of this link? It is known that p53 is activated by telomere wear and that, once activated; p53 suppresses PGC-1α and PGC-1β.

These molecules regulate the mitochondrial function and antioxidant protection.

So telomere shortening leads to activation of the p53 dependent *pathway* resulting in a disruption of mitochondrial function.

It is of particular interest that the researchers could establish that by restoring the telomerase gene the mitochondria including their function, number and antioxidant protection could be normalized.

With this it is unequivocally demonstrated that the mitochondria as a 'cause' of aging are wholly dependent on the telomeres.

In other words: aging is exclusively determined by the telomeres.[40]

However, the death-knell of the Free Radical Theory is not the Telomere Theory but the fact that, despite her 'top position' in the past 50 years, reduction of free radicals by antioxidant supplementation has not resulted in increasing (maximal) lifespan both in animals and man. This is fully discussed in a paper in the leading journal *Scientific American* under the telling tile **The Myth of Antioxidants** (February 2013). This does not mean that antioxidants are useless or unimportant, but the review article shows that the mitochondrial free radical theory is completely invalid as a theory of aging.

The Telomere Theory is *really* the only game in town and the fundamental role of telomerase has not only been shown in cell culture, but also in animal experiments (mouse), in which life extension between 25-50 percent could be achieved by activating telomerase.

Even of greater interest as 'proof of principle' is that scientists of the University of Nottingham (UK) have found that a certain type of flatworm can become immortal by maintenance of the telomerase enzyme.[41]

---

40 Sahin, E., et. al. Nature, 120, 470, 20, 2011.
41 Thomas, C.J. et.al. Telomeres maintenance and telomerase activity are differentially regulated in asexual and sexual worms, Proc. Nat. Ac. Sc. February 12, 2012.

This proves that telomerase is not only able to confer immortality to cells but also to organisms, from worm to man.

Chapter 23

Secondary causes of aging

The main secondary causes of aging are:

- **glycation**
- **free radicals**
- **inflammation**

Glycation
The concept 'glycation' was mentioned in chapters 5 and 7. To refresh your memory: glycation is the process by which sugars and proteins chemically combine (caramelizing). When this occurs in the kitchen (at high temperatures) a nice well-done steak or a lovely brownish omelette results.

Caramelizing outside the body (food) is called **exogenous** glycation (exogenous = outside the body) to distinguish it from caramelizing inside the body, the so-called **endogenous** glycation (endogenous = inside the body). The great danger of glycation is, however, certain very harmful end products referred to by the acronym AGEs (Advanced Glycation End products).

The term AGE, deliberately chosen, tells it all: AGEs (plural of AGE) cause aging! People used to think that AGEs in food were harmless. In the last 30 years we know better: they are very harmful.

About 30 percent of the AGEs in food is absorbed by the body and causes, via a process of 'chronic inflammation' in which the immune system is involved, serious damage over time, varying from atherosclerosis to cataract.

In order to show you how harmful glycation (AGEs) in food really is, I mention an experiment in mice, in which one group received the normal food and the other group food with 50 per cent less AGEs (same kind of food, but prepared at lower temperature and shorter cooking time).

The result? Mice who received 50 per cent less AGEs in their food lived on the average 15 per cent longer than those in the control group.[42]

Translated to humans it would mean that if all men in the West (Netherlands) would consume food with 50 percent less AGEs their life expectancy would rise from the current 80 years to 92.

As Wikipedia mentions tersely, AGEs are causally involved in maculae degeneration, cardiovascular diseases, type-2 diabetes and other chronic diseases and conditions.

> The official list of conditions and diseases caused or aggravated by AGEs is as follows:
>
> Alzheimer's disease
> cancer
> type-2 diabetes
> Atherosclerosis
> stroke, heart attack, aneurysm
> rheumatic conditions
> cataract & macular degeneration
> skin conditions

From the wealth of data I'll mention only one to give you some idea of the harmful effects of AGEs.

It has been found that in osteoarthritis, an inflammation that afflicts 15 percent of elderly people, the AGE substance pentosidine is found in high concentration in the affected cartilage and correlates (don't panic) with COMP[43], a biomarker of cartilage destruction.[44]

AGEs in food

The higher the temperature and the longer the cooking time the more AGEs. If you want to optimize your health it would be best

---
42   Cai, W. et.al. Am. J. Pathol. 170, 1893, 2007.
43   COMP=cartilage oligomeric matrix protein.
44   Senoit, A, et.al. Ann Reum Dis 64, 886, 2005.

to banish the frying pan and oven from your kitchen. Frying, roasting, etc. occur at temperatures of 160º or higher, while 100° C, the boiling temperature of water, is the least harmful.

(At high altitude the boiling point of water is 90° C, by which AGEs formation is only 1/3 of normal; indeed, owning a Chalet in Zermatt is highly recommended.)

With the exception of the rare health-conscious cook, like the mistress, the better the cook the more harmful the dish.

Generally speaking fried, grilled and roasted meat products (both red meat as well as chicken) contain the highest AGEs values, so, for this reason alone it is better to eat fish or a vegetarian diet and of course, avoid frying, etc., as much as possible, preferably using water (including steam). Unfortunately, nearly everything that's delicious or tasty, including wok, is less wholesome. Wok occurs at a high temperature and the delicious taste of vegetables and meat is the result of caramelizing, something we just want to avoid.

As I said it is better to eat fish rather than meat (including chicken) because fried fish has a much lower AGE-content than fried meat.

Instead of the oven or frying pan it is better to use the so-called crockpot or slow cook pan, which is very suitable to simmer meat very slowly at a temperature of 90^0 C (see google: crockpot).

Another safe way to prepare a tasty meat dish (and fish, tofu, etc.) is to marinate (with vinegar or some other acid). The high acidity insures that the AGEs formation is considerably lower. Marinade is an essential part of the Mediterranean diet, the most wholesome Western diet.

In order to give you an impression the frame below lists the AGEs content of a number of foodstuffs per portion, rounded off and expressed in the standard unit kU (don't worry).

Frankfurter	10.000
Hamburger	5.000
meat ball	5.000
chicken breast broiled	5.500
chicken nuggets	7.500
smoked salmon	500
cheese	2000-1000
egg (boiled)	200
ei (fried)	1.200
tofu (fried)	3.500
French fries	700
macaroni with cheese (oven)	4.000
toast sandwich (cheese)	4.500
oatmeal	50
apple	15

The daily AGEs intake is on the average about 15,000 kU. For optimal health over time it is desirable to keep this value below 5000. Above 20,000 the 'consequences of diabetes without diabetes' come into being over time. The complications of diabetes are mainly attributable to glycation and its end products, AGEs.

AGEs damage
One of the actions of AGEs is denaturing of body proteins and other giant molecules, including DNA. The most important component of connective tissue is collagen (a protein). AGEs cause collagen molecules to stick together, so-called cross-linking, resulting in networks, which for example, cause our skin (wrinkles) and arteries lose their elasticity.

Moreover the arteries become, just like an old windshield wiper, brittle and fragile, which increases the risk of a brain haemorrhage.

The loss of elasticity of the arterial wall results in (systolic) hypertension with all its attendant risks.

AGEs adhere to certain bindings spots in the cell wall, the so-called RAGEs (receptors for AGE), resulting in the activation of certain genes in the DNA, leading to an enormous increase of free radicals (up to 50 times) and an increase in inflammation (here an abnormal reaction of the immune system), resulting in a worsening of atherosclerosis.[45]

---

45 This occurs via activation of *NF-kB,* a critical factor in inflammation induction.

Since the increase in free radical production leads to an increase in AGEs, a vicious circle is created through which not only organs (kidneys, heart, skin, eyes) and the vascular system are affected, but the whole aging process is accelerated.

Cataract is the result of cross-linking of the *crystalline* proteins of the lens by AGEs. Kidney failure is a much-feared complication in diabetes patients and is the result of cross-linking of the proteins in the kidney filters (the glomeruli) by AGEs. But also without diabetes, just by a high AGEs intake via food this kidney damage may occur.

The lesson we should draw from all this misery is this:

AGEs are very dangerous and not only accelerate the aging process, but increase the risk of chronic conditions at a more advanced age.

For the rest, and this is inevitable, even at a low AGEs intake via food and a normal blood glucose level glycation will continue at a modest level due to both factors, so that glycation – even under ideal circumstances - contributes to the aging of our body.

Preventive measures

As I said cooking at low temperatures (100º C) is the best way to minimize glycation. Foodstuffs with a high AGEs content, such as meat products and processed meats (sausage, ham, etc.) should be avoided.

What misery: no luncheon meat, no fricandeau, no ham, no smoked-dry beef, roast beef, or salami. What then should I put on my bread, for Christ's sake? Jam (sugar) is bad, cheese is not too healthy either and meat products are taboo. Moreover bread (carbohydrates, see chapter 9) is not recommended.

Yes, it is indeed a big problem for Western man. My advice is: avoid meat products and jam and limit yourself to cheese, or, better marmite (bah!). Let me mention in passing to get you out of your depression, a little anecdote. As you know Marmite is a typical British eccentricity. During World War II the Marmite factory in Vauxhall, near London, was (accidentally) bombed by the Germans and destroyed. According to an ultra-secret report (I was one of the few with access to it) this led to demoralisation and great panic among the populace! Thanks to the personal intervention of Churchill, lover of gravy with a touch of marmite on his roast beef and Yorkshire pudding, the Marmite production was back to normal within weeks. Without Churchill's swift action England might have lost the war ...

Do agents exist to combat the harmful effects of AGEs?

Indeed, they do, although their effect is modest. Below is a list of natural substances and metformin:

1. benfotiamine, a fat-soluble form of thiamine, vitamin B2
2. pyrdoxamine, a variant of pyridoxine or vitamin B6
3. vitamin C
4. alpha-lipoic acid
5. carnosine
6. resveratrol
7. curcumin
8. metformin

With the exception of benfotiamine and pyridoxamine these substances are discussed elsewhere in this book.

Finally the question, "Are their safe agents available to repair existing damage (cross-linking, etc.)?"

Unfortunately the answer is no, perhaps with the exception of the drug alagebrium that is able to repair existing cross-linking in animals. Alas, it has thus far (2014) not been able to meet FDA's strict standards.

Obviously keeping your blood glucose level low (metformin, etc.) is just as important to prevent glycation.

Free radicals

Free radicals are as destructive as a shower of sparks. But what is a free radical? In order to really understand it you should almost be a chemist.

All you should know is presented below. And remember, 'Knowledge is power'. Here power over your own body and your life.

An atom is like the solar system, with electrons, like planets, circling the minute nucleus in the centre.

Atoms and molecules have (don't be alarmed) 2 electrons in a path (orbit), just as some planets have two moons. It is called 'paired electrons'. But when there is only one electron in the path (unpaired) disaster looms. For the atom (molecule) cries out for 2 electrons (the normal state) and the atom (molecule) steals an electron from the neighbouring bio-molecule (protein, DNA) to restore the initial condition (2 electrons). An atom or molecule with an unpaired electron is called a free radical and is because of its 'avidity' very aggressive and dangerous.

A bio-molecule (protein, etc.) with 1 electron (in orbit) is a damaged molecule. This damages the cell. One of the best-known actions of free radicals is damage to cell membranes as a result of a process known as lipid peroxidation (fats turning rancid).

This *peroxidation* (turning rancid) of fats in the cell membrane results in hardening of the membrane (the skin of the cell), diminished permeability, diminished activity of the membrane enzymes and membrane receptors (such as hormone receptors and RAGEs (see above).

By damaging the cells the aging process is accelerated, as well as progression to cancer, cardiovascular diseases and other aging diseases, including diabetes and Alzheimer disease.

> **Free radical**
> An atom or group of atoms with at least one unpaired electron. In the body this is often an oxygen molecule that has lost an electron and wants to stabilize itself by stealing an electron from a nearby molecule.

Background
The father of the free radical theory is the American chemist and physician Denham Harman, who was employed as a research scientist at Shell in the fifties where he acquired 30 patents in his name, among which a patent for plastic strips to kill flies. Even

then he was greatly interested in the process of aging, which inspired him to study medicine at Stanford University (Cal.). His brilliant idea that free radicals play a significant role in aging and aging diseases was inspired by the fact that X-rays are so dangerous because of the creation of the very aggressive hydroxyl-radical from the water molecule H_2O. (Our body consists for 60 per cent of water by weight).

Too much oxygen also acts via the same mechanism: the formation of the hydroxyl-radical. In the past premature babies received too much extra oxygen, resulting in blindness by the overproduction of free radicals attacking the crystalline proteins of the eye lens.

Madame Curie died young from aplastic anaemia as a result of radiation, but was already blind from cataract and suffered from cancer and bone marrow exhaustion effects of too much radioactive radiation and, so, of free radical overload.

During the production of energy in the cell's power stations, the mitochondria (see chapter 7), where oxygen is used for the cell's 'respiration', 1 to 2 percent of the oxygen is converted into a so-called oxygen radical. Via this radical, called the superoxide-radical, the hydroxyl–radical is formed.

So, our own cell respiration produces exactly the same harmful radical as X-ray radiation.

In order to put the fear of God into you I mention that each body cell produces about 4 million hydroxyl–radicals daily. Although a high percentage is neutralized by the body's own antioxidants and affected proteins, fats and DNA's are partially replaced by the cell, it should be clear that our trillions of body cells will suffer a lot of damage from free radicals in the course of a lifetime, thus accelerating the aging process.

An interesting fact that lends support to Harman's theory is the link between the lifespan of a species and the level of antioxidants, the protection against free radicals. The longer the lifespan the higher the level of antioxidants, including the body's own enzyme catalase.

The substances that neutralize free radicals are (called) antioxidants.

Experiments by Harman and others in mice and other test animals have shown that adding extra antioxidants (like vitamin C, vitamin E and lipoic acid) slows down aging and increases the **mean** lifespan.

The criterion of the REAL cause of aging is, however, that manipulating this 'presumed cause' results in an increase in the **maximum** lifespan of the species (so, for man, from 120 to-say-150 years).

This has never been achieved with antioxidants. From this it follows that free radicals are not the fundamental cause of aging, but only, just as X-ray radiation, smoking (huge source of free radicals) and chronic inflammation, accelerate the aging process.

The most important antioxidants that protect us against free radicals are discussed in a separate chapter.

A definition

I end this section presenting a term we'll meet again later: **oxidative stress.**

The opponents of free radicals are, as mentioned, the antioxidants, substances our body produces itself (like the enzyme catalase) or are ingested (vitamins C and E, flavonoids, etc.).

If the antioxidant protection is inadequate an imbalance exists which is referred to by the term **oxidative stress.**

Inflammation

The significance of chronic low-grade inflammation follows from the finding that it is involved in at least seven of the leading causes of death in the West: heart disease, cancer, stroke, Alzheimer disease, kidney failure and atherosclerosis. It also plays a significant role in aging, in the sense that it accelerates and aggravates the process.

But what is inflammation really?

We have to make a clear distinction between **acute** inflammation and **chronic** inflammation. We are all familiar with acute inflammation: an infected finger (felon) is the classic example. In medical textbooks acute inflammation is characterized by the familiar 4 symptoms: redness, heat, swelling and pain. But of course not in the vulgar English tongue, but in Latin: *rubor, calor, tumor and dolor.* This inflammation as a reaction to a trauma or infection serves to remove damaged tissue (cells), and to kill bacteria. White blood cells of the immune system are always involved. You might say: acute inflammation is a reaction of the immune system (lymphocytes, etc.) to trauma or infection. It is an effective response of the body.

Chronic inflammation is, however, something different altogether: it is very harmful in the long run.

Chronic inflammation is almost always the result of the presence of defective cells and instead of promoting health it leads to disease and accelerated aging.

The most familiar form of chronic inflammation is rheumatism (rheumatoid arthritis) (red, swollen, hot and painful knee) and these patients have a decreased life expectancy.

But the far milder forms of chronic inflammation (like atherosclerosis) are, just as the 'silent condition' hypertension very harmful, since they accelerate the aging process and play a causal role in life threatening aging diseases.

Yes, but you will say, the 'silent condition' hypertension can be established with a tonometer, though it is 'silent'. But how do you determine chronic low-grade inflammation? Formerly by means of the erythrocyte sedimentation rate (ESR), currently by a much more sensitive blood test, the C-reactive protein (CRP) test. This test is greatly elevated in rheumatism and to a lesser degree in severe forms of atherosclerosis. Just like cholesterol, etc. it is a bio-marker for heart conditions and heart attacks, since chronic inflammation greatly increases the risk of a heart attack. A very sensitive variant of the CRP test is the newer *high-sensitive* CRP, or hs-CRP, that together with total cholesterol and HDL-cholesterol constitutes a strong predictor of future trouble in apparently healthy persons, because low-grade chronic inflammation (vessel wall) plays an important role in the development of atherosclerosis.

In passing it may be mentioned that statins like Lipitor, are not protective because of lowering cholesterol, but just as aspirin, because of their inflammation inhibiting properties. But fish oil (safe and healthy) inhibits inflammation as well and should be the first choice, although BIG PHARMA can make no money from it and so it is not prescribed by doctors. Yes, that's the way medicine works.

Causes of low-grade chronic inflammation
The impatient reader may skip this section, but for a clear understanding of the relationship between the 'big three', glycation, free radicals and inflammation it makes sense not to skip this section.

1 Leaking mitochondria
A damaged cell attracts, just like a bacteria, white blood cells (immune reaction). The cell damage is often the result of the increased production of free radicals (shower of sparks) in the mitochondria (power plants) associated with aging. As I said before, mitochondria may be compared with the black pits of a kiwi. Each cell has 500-1000 mitochondria. As a result of this increase of free radicals the cell membrane (the 'skin' of the cell) becomes permeable, leading to substances leaking out of the mitochondrium (single) to the environment, the inside of the cell, called the *cytoplasm*, the fluid in which the mitochondria are 'floating'.

This contains so-called *Pattern recognition receptors (PRR's) that* normally initiate an immune reaction against intracellular germs (virus, bacteria). But the molecules from the mitochondrion are interpreted as 'foreign', so PRR's also activate an immune response, with the white blood cells swinging into action to attack the 'infected' cell and destroy it. Result: local invasion of white blood cells (inflammation) and cell death. Mind you: here the free radicals are in fact the cause of the inflammation.

> After detection of the potential threat the PRR's form a complex called inflammasome, which activates the inflammation cytokine *interleukin-1b*, which recruits the components of the immune system to destroy the 'infected cell'.*
>
> * Tschopp, Mitochondria, Sovereign of inflammation? Eur. J. Immun.41, 1196, 2011.

2 Oxidised cholesterol
This is mainly involved in atherosclerosis, which is in essence an inflammation process. The well-known LDL-cholesterol, better known as the 'bad' cholesterol may precipitate in the artery wall when the blood level is elevated. By a number of factors it can be oxidised locally (in the vessel wall) or earlier in the bloodstream, when it reacts with free radicals. This oxy-LDL attracts inflammatory cells of the immune system, among which (don't be alarmed) macrophages (a kind of white blood cells). These cells goggle up cholesterol, making them look under the microscope like foam-filled cells, from which the name foam cells derives. This is the beginning of the much-feared plaque of atherosclerosis. Dead foam cells produce substances that induce the smooth muscle cells to multiply. The plaque or atheroma is a pustule filled with matter consisting of foam cells, cholesterol crystals, smooth muscle cells and other junk (see chapter 17).

Conclusion: oxidised LDL-cholesterol (oxy-LDL) is the cause of the later stages of atherosclerosis, a process of chronic inflammation.

3 AGEs
AGEs (see above) can also cause inflammation through the following mechanism. As we have discussed earlier AGEs can stick to certain 'antennae' in the cell membrane called RAGEs (receptors for advanced glycation products).

This sends a signal to DNA in the cell nucleus by means of (don't be alarmed) a molecule with the difficult name *nuclear factor kappa-B* (NF-kB) that enters the nucleus and activates a large number of inflammation genes. This alerts the immune system and initiates a local inflammation reaction, in which of course white blood cells are involved.

So, here we see that AGEs (glycation) can activate inflammation.

Between the 3 secondary causes of aging, glycation, free radicals and inflammation, a close interaction exists, resulting in a vicious circle that accelerates the aging process. A discussion of this must however be omitted. As had been mentioned in the discussion of glycation AGEs cause chronic inflammation and the binding of AGE to RAGE (AGE receptor) induces free radical production and inflammation. Conversely, free radicals activate the formation of AGEs. One big tangle. Enough to drive you crazy!

I end this chapter with the following quote: 'AGEs are free radical boosters; they are usually formed by free radicals and subsequently exert their toxic actions by producing more free radicals, thereby causing *oxidative stress* and thus inflammation". Truly, a labyrinth.

Measures to decrease chronic inflammation
I only mention the following:

- metformin
- aspirin (not recommended)
- statins (not recommended)
- exercise
- vitamin E (this is especially effective against the oxidation of cholesterol in the vessel wall)
- resveratrol
- fish oil
- Co-enzyme Q10
- losing weight (the heavier the more inflammation)
- stress avoidance

Technical note

The role of DNA methylation in aging will not be discussed. It is a mine field, while it is moreover not clear whether it is a causal factor in aging of an epiphenomenon, like grey hair. For a recent review see A.A. Johnson et al. 'The Role of Methylation in Aging, Rejuvenation and Age-related Disease', Rejuvenation Research, 15, 483, 2012

Chapter 24

The most important anti-aging antioxidants

In chapter 23 the three main secondary causes of aging were discussed: glycation, free radicals and inflammation.

As we have seen there is a close interaction between these 3 factors, whereby free radicals occupy a key position.

The opponents of free radicals, the defenders of our body, are the antioxidants that neutralize the free radicals.

As I mentioned in chapter 23, when the antioxidants are too weak in relation to free radicals (analogy: police too weak in relation to mafia) it is called **oxidative stress**.

Oxidative because most free radicals in the body contain the oxygen atom.

Oxidative stress, not free radicals per se, is a very important factor in aging and its consequences.

With aging (after 50) the overload by free radicals increases because 1) the mitochondria (power plants) are no longer functioning properly and so produce more free radicals and 2) the production of the body's own antioxidants like glutathione and catalase (enzyme) decreases. Result: more oxidative stress, which accelerates aging and thus creates a vicious circle.

The following sounds a bit 'abstract' (obscure), but since your health and your life are determined by the degree of oxidative stress I urge you to read the next section attentively. It is very important.

The antioxidant network
Our body has at its disposal a so-called antioxidant network consisting of vitamin C, vitamin E, co-enzyme Q10 (produced in the liver), alpha lipoic acid (in vegetables, etc.) and glutathione.

The essence of this network is that the antioxidants functionally restore one another. Here is an example.

When vitamin E disarms a free radical, it becomes itself a weak free radical. But unlike the bad free radicals the vitamin E–radical can be recycled, that is restored to an antioxidant, by means of vitamin C.

Chemically very complex, but all you and I should know is that the components of such a network cooperate closely, increasing the protective action against free radicals enormously. Such 'amplifying' cooperation is called synergy, a concept that may sound familiar to you.

The following supplements constitute the antioxidant network:
vitamin C, vitamin E, co-enzyme Q10, lipoic acid and ginkgo biloba.

A personal note: it goes without saying that I'm taking these preparations daily.

Before proceeding it is relevant to point out that the antioxidant network was discovered by professor Lester Packer and his team at Berkeley University in California (Robert Oppenheimer's *alma mater*). Professor Packer's laboratory is the Mecca of scientists in this field and the mere fact that the Packer laboratory bears his name bears witness to his super status as a scientist.

At the time I also had my own laboratory at Leyden University, which to my chagrin has never been allowed to bear my name.

Very briefly I shall discuss some aspects of these substances using the highly recommended book *The Antioxidant Miracle* by Lester Packer.

Vitamin C
Vitamin C is a powerful free radical fighter and is essential for a strong immune system. Studies have shown that people who take extra vitamin C supplements live longer and enjoy better health than others.

Vitamin E
Vitamin E is fat-soluble and is transported in the bloodstream by lipoproteins (like LDL and HDL), where it protects cholesterol against oxidation by free radicals.

Oxidized cholesterol (oxy-cholesterol), not cholesterol per se, is the cause of blood vessel inflammation, and thus atherosclerosis. Vitamin E protects against heart diseases and Alzheimer's disease.

Co-enzyme Q10
Co-enzyme Q10 is fat-soluble and acts synergistically with vitamin E in the antioxidant cycle to protect the cell against free radical damage. A large number of studies have shown that Co-Q10 is effective in the treatment of heart failure, angina pectoris and hypertension.

Lipoic acid
Lipoic acid (full name: alpha-lipoic acid) is very important because it boosts the production of the body's most important (own) antioxidant glutathione. Orally glutathione is not absorbed, which is a pity as the glutathione level is a measure for the health of the organism. An example: a study in the Lancet (the leading British medical journal) had shown that the glutathione level is very low in hospital patients, low in policlinic patients, high in young people and low in the elderly (above 70 the glutathione level is more than 30 percent lower than at an earlier age) and in patients with a geriatric disease. At every age a low glutathione level is associated with premature death. The rule is: the higher your glutathione level the better you're protected.

The most effective way to increase your glutathione level is the use of alpha-glutathione, which by the way, has a molecular structure similar to that of glutathione.

Lipoic acid is present in food, but only in minimal amounts. So you would have to eat 3 kilo's spinach for 1 mg lipoic acid, while the effective dose to increase the glutathione level is 100 mg a day.

Ginkgo biloba

Ginkgo biloba is a powerful antioxidant, especially in use to improve memory.

A patient of mine told me that his memory had considerably improved after using gingko biloba for a few months. He interpreted my facial expression mistakenly and burst out angrily,
"You don't believe me? My wife can affirm it. Etc." For me such an outburst is evidence that it worked.

But here it is not about memory, but only about ginkgo biloba's role in the Packer antioxidant network.

Before discussing the theme 'dosage' just a note about the action of synergy (increased combined action of a number of factors).
You don't need to know anything about electronics to grasp the following analogy.
Suppose you have three sound amplifiers. Each of them amplifies the sound ten times.
If you put them in parallel you obtain an amplification of 10+10+10 =30.
But if you connect them in series (one after the other) the amplification is 10x10x10 = 1000.
This is an example of 'synergy', not a sum, but a multiplication of the individual actions.

That's how the antioxidant network of vitamin C, vitamin E, lipoic acid and gingko biloba works.

Dosage

The dosages required for the antioxidant network are relatively low.
An example: as we saw in chapter 16 it makes sense to take several grams of vitamin C in divided doses for e.g. strengthening of the collagen in the vessel wall.
But for the network 500 mg vitamin C (divided over two portions) is sufficient. The same holds for vitamin E, lipoic acid, etc.

Here is a simplified version of the so-called Packer plan:

Twice daily:	Vitamin E	200 mg
	Vitamin C	250 mg
	Co-Q10	30 mg
	Lipoic acid	50 mg
	Ginkgo biloba	30 mg

You can, of course, buy these supplements separately. Via typing *Antioxidant Network* or www.networkantioxidants.com you obtain the right combination and dosages professor Packer recommends. This is also cheaper.

Personally, I, of course, use the Packer preparations, however supplemented with higher doses of C, E and Co-Q10.

The serious student of aging is strongly advised to study professor Packer's book The Antioxidant Miracle.

Antioxidants and AGE's
Let me end this section with the following quote from professor Packer's book (abbr.)

'Antioxidants can also prevent another well-known aging-promoter, the formation of AGEs [see chapter 23]. The universal antioxidant lipoic acid, as well as the other antioxidants, can slow down the formation of AGE, which in the long run can have a huge impact on every organ system in the body, from skin (wrinkles), lentil senilis ('old-age spots'), to cataract and heart disease.'

Glutathione: the main antioxidant in our body

Keep your glutathione level high. Low glutathione values are a harbinger of illness and premature death.
Lipoic acid increases the glutathione level.
N-acetyl L-cystein (NAC), too, increases the glutathione level, but to a far lesser degree than lipoic acid.

Glutathione has - apart from its function as an antioxidant - other actions.
An example: if DNA is damaged, certain enzymes are required to repair it. Glutathione activates these enzymes in DNA damage.

Some more functions of glutathione:

- It plays (in the liver) a central role in detoxification. Via a process called (don't worry) *S-conjugation* it binds to the poison, enabling it to be excreted by the kidneys.
- It strengthens the immune system. People with low glutathione levels have a weakened immune system.
- Glutathione is considered an anti-aging antioxidant and rightly so.
- Example: in mosquitos an increase of the glutathione content by 50 percent by adding NAC (N-acetyl cysteine) results in a life-extension of 40 percent. In the fruit fly (a good model for man) by 26 percent.

Important:
Currently glutathione can be given orally in the form of acetyl-glutathione (see google); effective, but expensive.

Chapter 25

Diabetes and insulin therapy

This mini-chapter only deals with type-2 diabetes, the diabetes after middle age, which is often associated with overweight.

Although the disease is often progressive and can lead to a total loss of insulin production (only then insulin therapy is inevitable), administering insulin is in most cases the least attractive option for the patient, quite apart from the needle. In a nutshell, the best treatment is: 1) **minimal consumption of carbohydrates, 2) a relatively low-calorie diet and 3) metformin.**

Let me begin with an anecdote from a distant past.

As a youth I heard in the Japanese concentration camp in Java a professor sighing dejectedly, "We have no insulin, this means death for hundreds of diabetes patients ..."

I worked in the sickbay at the time and both my own observations as well as the statistics showed that the men with diabetes type-2 remained relatively healthy (without insulin or other medicines). The secret: there was little to eat.

The second anecdote is taken from the book *The Food Hourglass* by the Belgian doctor Kris Verburgh (see chapter 6). It starts with an introductory remark:

> I had always been taught that diabetes type-2 was a chronic disease: incurable. And that people, once they start injecting insulin must always keep injecting. Great was my amazement when I read the first reports about diabetes patients who no longer ate bread, potatoes, pasta and rice and lost weight considerably. After a few weeks they had not only lost many kilograms, they no longer

had to inject insulin. I have observed similar results in my own diabetes patients. The first was an uncle of mine when I was still a medical student. I advised him to refrain from eating bread, potatoes, pasta and rice. He injected himself three times daily with insulin for years and despite frantic dietary attempts his weight kept increasing, as well as his blood pressure and eye problems. But by not eating bread, pasta, rice and potatoes any more he not only lost a spectacular amount of weight; after a few weeks he didn't need to use insulin any more: his blood sugar levels stayed normal.

The fact that patients can drastically reduce their insulin use by following this diet is very interesting. Although you can't live without insulin [most patients still produce their own insulin in the pancreas, J.D.], insulin is a double-edged sword for diabetics.

Insulin has, just as IGF ['insulin-like growth factor, J.D.] a growth hormone–like action. Insulin makes most individuals gain weight. But weight gain is exactly the greatest risk factor in diabetes. In short, every diabetes patient who injects insulin is caught in a vicious circle: the insulin makes him heavier, aggravating his diabetes, requiring more insulin, gaining more weight. Etc. (unquote)

The adverse effects of insulin excess are discussed in chapters 1-6.

In his book *Fantastic Voyage* (with Terry Grossman, MD) about life-extension Raymond Kurzweil, genius and polyhistor, who designed the speech computer for professor Hawking (of wheelchair fame) tells the following personal story:

> When I turned 35 I got diabetes type 2 [family condition]
> I received the conventional treatment with insulin, but this made matters worse by causing considerable weight gain, which in its turn created an apparent need for more insulin. My personal quest let to a number of ideas about health that enabled me to get off insulin and keep my di-

abetes under control, simply by diet, exercise and stress management.

He further writes:

> To overcome my type-2 diabetes I use chrome and metformin (a powerful anti-aging drug that reduces insulin resistance and that we recommend for everyone older than 50.)

These were 3 anecdotal examples. As you have seen in chapters 1-6 insulin is adding fuel to the fire. As boss over your own body instead of your doctor's serf you as a diabetes patient should try to do everything to get off insulin. There are other options, of which metformin is the most interesting. Unless your pancreas doesn't produce any insulin at all, of course.

My advice is:
Virtually no carbohydrates from bread, potatoes, pasta and rice, a calorie-restricted diet, metformin (this also reduces the sense of hunger), sufficient exercise and no insulin.

Chapter 26

Are we our brain?

In 2012 the wonderful book of the renowned brain researcher professor Swaab appeared (in Dutch), titled: **We are our brain**.

Although it is outside the field of neuroscience, professor Swaab arrives at the conclusion, as suggested by the title, that we're nothing but our brain. Our brain dies, so we die. Swaab says: "When we die, our brain stops functioning and nothing is left of mind. Dead is dead, nothing can be done about it."

This conclusion is diametrically opposed to that of the cardiologist Dr. Pim van Lommel, author of the hugely popular book **Consciousness Beyond Life,** which, on the basis of scientific studies on NDE's (Near-Death-Experiences) published in leading medical journals like THE LANCET, argues that the mind ('soul') is separate from the brain and so you continue to exist after death and are in fact 'immortal'.

Since this book is about life extension, it is only natural to pay attention to the burning existential question, "Is there life after death?", or is death literally and figuratively the black hole?

Let us start from a virgin sheet of paper.

Suppose there is a conscious, interesting life after death and you believe that dead is dead.

For many - not for all - not a cheerful thought. What a pity! A feast awaits you and you're expecting a dungeon.

Conversely, suppose dead is indeed dead, but you believe in the continued existence of the soul, in a shining hereafter. Then you face the future in confidence since you 'know' that death is only the transition to a different kind of existence, even if it is only a delusion.

These were two silly reflections with a grain of truth.

But now to the point. The evidence in Dr. van Lommel's book is for me, physician–biologist, amateur psychical researcher and thinker, convincing, but some readers of both above-mentioned books (Schwaab and Van Lommel) would still remain 'agnostic', torn between 'hope and fear', heaven and a black hole.

Life or no life after death: am I my brain or not ?
It is my intention to convince you in one blow that the mind (personality, spirit) continues to exist after death. I'll explain it in brief: less than two pages.

Ah, Defares will never manage, I can hear you think. If Dr. van Lommel, after hundreds of pages of empirical evidence, fails to convince me, how could Defares manage to pull it off? *No way*!

Oh, yes, I'll manage, because I'll make use of the absolutely unique case from parapsychology, the aftermath of the disaster of the British airship (zeppelin) R101, that crashed at the French coast on its maiden voyage from London to India in 1930.

Fasten your seatbelts and listen to a fantastic but true story that proves the continued existence of the personality beyond a shadow of a doubt. The next text is taken from my earlier book **Beyond the Borders of this Life.**

The disaster of airship R101
On October 4 1939 the British airship R101 on its maiden flight to India crashed near a hill at Beauvais, France. 48 of the 54 passengers lost their lives. This scandalous disaster was the result of official intrigues, undue political pressures to meet an unrealistic deadline and gross technological blunders.

On October 6 1939 a scientifically designed séance was held, in which, among others, the well-known parapsychologist Harry Price, the journalist Ian. D. Coster and the very talented young medium Eileen Garrett [generally regarded as the most important and gifted medium of the 20th century] were present. The purpose of the session was to contact the recently deceased British novelist and spiritualist Sir Conan Doyle. Instead of making contact with the creator of Sherlock Holmes, an anxious voice came through of an entity that called itself lieutenant H. Carmichael Irwin. This turned out to be the name of the captain of the R101.

The voice provided highly technical details about the course and the causes of the disaster.

The journalist wrote an article in the Morning Post over this, which came to the attention of engineer Dr. Charlton, who was closely associated with the construction of the R101. After studying the séance report which he had obtained from Dr. Price he and his colleagues called it 'an amazing report', which contained over 20 classified technical details about the disaster. But there is more.

Major Olivier Villiers of the British Ministry of Civil Aviation and one of the members of the Court of Inquiry participated with others in a séance of Eileen Garrett. She is one of those rare mediums in whom, in trance, the voice (intonation, timbre, etc.) of the deceased person comes through.

Via the medium major Villiers was able to conduct a conversation with the (putative) captain and other deceased crew members, among whom pilot Scott. A fragment of this conversation between Villiers and Scott is presented below:

Villiers: "What was the matter? Irvin mentioned the nose of the airship?"

Scott: "Yes, problems with girders and engines."

Villiers: "I want to know exactly. Can you tell me where precisely? The longitudinal girders are numbered A to G."

Scott: "The uppermost is 0. Then downward A, B, C, etc. Look at the drawing. It was about the starboard side of 5C. When we returned from our second flight we saw that the girder was twisted, although not cracked, which led to problems with the covering ..." (Major Villiers then asked whether the girder was later broken and had pierced the covering.)

Scott: "No, not broken, torn. A huge rent on the starboard side of 5C produced an abnormal pressure which forced us to do a nose dive. The pressure on the gas tanks was tremendous. Because of the outside pressure and the fact that de gas valve was to weak, the gas valve was simply blown away. At the same time the escaping gas ignited because of the fire from the engine's exhaust."

The subsequent judicial investigation showed that these and scores of other data agreed with the reconstruction.

It is almost superfluous to note that the medium was completely ignorant about aviation technology.

Especially the fact that via the 'conversation' between Villiers and the (putative) Scott a number of technical details came to light that were unknown to anyone alive at the time of the séance, offers strong support for the survival theory, since telepathy can't provide an alternative explanation in this case. Forty years later, in 1970, the parapsychologist Dr. A. Jarman, who in the late thirties had written his 455 page book about this event, wrote, "It is the technical aspect of this affair which makes this event unique in the history of spiritual phenomena. And I mean 'really' unique."

Indeed, qua evidential value this case is unique.

It proves with compelling logic the continued existence of the personality (*you*) after death.

On the internet you'll find hundreds of pages (including Wikipedia) devoted to this unique case: google 'R101' and you will be swamped.

If you're by now not convinced of the reality of life after this life and the continuity of the personality after death, then nothing can convince you.[46]

---

46   John Fuller. *The airmen who wouldn't die,* Putman, 1979.
    This is an exhaustive chronicle of the events.

Chapter 27

Meditation and aging

Let me start with two personal anecdotes. In the sixties my wife and I were great friends with Rita Meier, a woman in her early thirties who meditated a lot. Not like someone who practices Yoga or Transcendental Meditation, but serious stuff at Tibetan level: at least three hours a day and regularly studying under the guidance of Tibetan monks, both in Tibet and in Europe.

Thirty years later, after having lost sight of each other, I happened to meet her again in a gallery in Leyden. She was 65.

I was amazed: she looked like a woman of 40 with a youthful aura to boot. By the way, I was accompanied by my new medical assistant, Angela, 22, as some of her boyfriend's works were on exhibition there. Suddenly I heard someone calling behind me, "Hey, James, dirty old man, is there life in the old dog yet ..." It was Rita.

At a parents' meeting a psychologist, a Maharishi Mahesh Yogi follower, gave a lecture on – according to him - the scientifically established positive influence of Transcendental Meditation on aging: people would stay much younger than their chronological age, he claimed. I was sceptical.

But, later I read the trailblazing paper of Dr. Robert Wallace in *the International Journal of Neuroscience* (16, 53, 1982) on the influence of Transcendental Meditation on aging. Dr. Wallace found that people with an average age of 50 who had been practising TM for five years or longer had an average biological age which was 12 years younger than their chronological age. This means that (on the average) a 55-year old meditator is biologically 43.

Some subjects who had meditated for a very long time (up to 30 years) even had a biological age that was 27 years younger. A 65-years-old with a biological age of 38!

Since, scores of scientific studies have been published on this subject confirming this conclusion.

Rita, my friend, 65, with a biological age of 38? My fleeting impression seemed to confirm this possibility.

But before proceeding just a little comment. Meditation to stay 'young and healthy' is a piece of cake. Yogi's from India and Tibet meditate to reach the state of *Samadhi* (Enlightenment), a mighty endeavour. Meditation for our purpose is very simple, as Dr. Herbert Benson of Harvard shows in his book *The Relaxation Response.*

Just sit relaxed, close your eyes and don't worry about thoughts drifting like clouds in your mental space. This lack of concern is called *Mindfulness*. You can focus you attention on your breathing, and repeat a mantra in silence (doesn't matter which, from 'Aum' to 'One' or 'Cola' and start for 5 minutes twice a day. The normal duration is 15 minutes, twice daily. You may even open your eyes to look at your watch. It is that simple.

But how can such a simple routine have any effect on your state of health, you may wonder.

Scientific studies have shown that it works.

These are the minimum instructions:

- Find a quiet spot.
- Sit down and relax your muscles, starting with your feet en ending at your face (facial muscles).
- Pay attention to your breathing and repeat a mantra with each breath.
- If you skip a mantra, not to worry.
- Let your thoughts drift like clouds.
- Continue for 15 minutes.

Yes, that's all, but as professor Benson has shown this simple exercise results in slowing down the process of aging.

But, since as we know from chapter 13, the telomere is the time clock of aging, and the rate of telomere shrinkage is the fundamental cause of aging, it is of great interest to discuss the findings concerning the effect of meditation on telomere shrinkage.

Meditation and telomeres
Regular meditation slows down the shrinkage of our telomeres to a considerable extent. This means that meditation is able to slow down the aging process at its most fundamental level (since telomere shortening is the cause of aging (chapter 13).

This has been shown by a study about the relation between meditation and telomeres by the Nobel laureate Elizabeth Blackburn and the psychologist Dr. E. Epel published in 2009 under the telling title **Can meditation slow rate of cellular aging? Cognitive stress, mindfulness and telomeres** (Ann.N.Y.Acad.Sci, 1172, 34, 2009).

It is saying a lot that professor Blackburn (who leads a more busy life than a Nobel prize winner?) has started meditating herself as a result of the outcome of this research.

This study has shown at a fundamental level how meditation can keep you much younger than your (chronological) age.

Meditate twice daily and you'll reap the harvest today and tomorrow.

Chapter 28

Smoking, a deadly sin

Although it is almost unthinkable that the reader of this book smokes, I will, just to make sure, devote a page to the evils of smoking.

Smoking is about the worst thing you can do to your body, so, to yourself.
Are you aspiring to a poor quality of life and a short lifespan, then, do smoke. It is that simple.

Smokers live on the average 10-18 years shorter and smoking is a big risk factor for heart attacks, strokes and cancer.

According to the trailblazing study involving 15,000 British doctors, at least half of life-long smokers die as a result of smoking. Another statistic: smokers have a 3 times greater risk of dying before sixty than non-smokers.

Just a personal observation. At the physiology laboratory in Leyden where I worked for ten years, there were two very heavy smokers, professor Duyff, the director, and Dr. Van Zanten, a young physicist. They smoked at least 2 packs a day. Professor Duyff died at 53 from lung cancer and Dr. Van Zanten at 42 from the same disease.

Of course, smoking also greatly increases the risk of other cancers, including kidney cancer, throat cancer, oesophagus cancer, bladder cancer, breast cancer and pancreas cancer.

Smoking is the main cause of severe atherosclerosis (narrowing of the arteries), resulting in angina pectoris (due to narrowing of the coronary arteries) and claudicatio intermittens (pain in the legs while walking, sometimes limiting the distance to yards). Most patients being treated for narrowed arteries in the chelation clinics (chapter 35) are heavy smokers.

But within the scope of this book the main message is that smoking greatly accelerates the aging process by accelerating at least two secondary causes of aging (chapter 23): free radicals (oxidative stress) and chronic inflammation. Free radicals also accelerate the shortening of the telomeres, the fundamental cause of aging.

The life-long smoker can be recognized by his looks: greyish skin, wrinkled, with the typical 'smokers face', as described many years ago in TIME magazine in a leading article on smoking.
Worth mentioning is a Swedish study of 300 women who had been judged 'attractive' when they were young.
Half of them were smokers. Their pictures were evaluated at middle age by a panel of middle-age men.
80 Percent of the non-smokers were judged as still 'attractive' and of the smokers less than 10 percent. How can this be? Greatly accelerated aging plus chronic 'poisoning'. When you're old on the inside, you're old on the outside and conversely, for (this is in German) as Goethe wrote long ago, "*Nichts ist innen, nichts ist außen, denn was drinnen ist, ist draußen .*"
Still smoking? Stop today or make the decision to stop, with or without the aid of a nicotine plaster.

Chapter 29

Losing weight: fast and permanent

Staying at your ideal weight is not a matter of following a weight loss diet (Atkins, etc.), but a matter of eating differently. Fortunately it is healthy and slows down aging to boot. It is eating according to the guidelines in chapter 2 and chapter 9: no bread, potatoes, pasta and rice (you may cheat). As an introduction I quote this passage taken from Kris Verburgh's excellent book **The Food Sandglass,** to which I referred before.

While discussing the theme of diabetes type-2 he writes (as quoted earlier):

"Great was my surprise when I read the first reports on diabetes patients who did no longer eat bread, potatoes, pasta and rice and lost considerable weight. I have seen similar results in my own diabetes patients. The first was an uncle of mine when I was still a medical student. I advised him to stop eating bread, potatoes, pasta and rice. He had been injecting himself for years with insulin and despite frantic dietary attempts his weight kept increasing, as well as his blood pressure and eye problems. Naturally he had to inject ever more insulin. But by no more eating bread, paste, rice and potatoes he didn't only lose a spectacular amount of weight, after a few weeks he didn't have to use insulin anymore: his blood sugar levels stayed normal. "(unquote).

Good grief, what for heaven's sake has an insulin patient to do with losing weight? you may wonder irritably.

Well, in the first place diabetes is nothing but accelerated ('enlarged') aging, the process that affects us all.

But more to the point: avoiding carbohydrates acts not only in diabetics, but also in normal healthy people as has been shown empirically. This is in fact the secret of the effectiveness of the Atkins diet: its secret is not the extra protein, but the avoidance of carbohydrates. Keeping slim for most people over 40 requires the elimination of these foods (once more: bread, potatoes, pasta and rice).

Oatmeal is allowed because of the low glycaemic index (see chapter 9).

You may take the Paleo-anti-aging diet as discussed in chapter 2 as a guideline to stay slim forever.

Mediterranean salads with beans, walnuts, avocado, tuna or eggs for lunch (with for example one slice of rye bread with cheese or fruit) and in the evening vegetables (carrots, broccoli, spinach, etc.) with beans (one medium potato is allowed as a concession) and as protein source fish, chicken or eggs. Why is the avoidance of carbohydrates so effective? An important reason is that with this diet the insulin levels stay low and insulin fattens, as is discussed in the earlier chapters.

***

Since this is not a treatise about weight loss, but a supplement to what has been discussed in earlier chapters, I'll end this chapter with an almost playful question.

"How many eggs a day may I consume?"

"At most 2 eggs a week, stupid! Every doctor will tell you that."

Baloney! The world's greatest authority on fats, cholesterol and health, the American biochemist professor M.G. Enig, says in her book **Know your Fats** that you can safely eat 12 eggs a day. In her book she offers a biochemical explanation for this striking statement, in which the so-called negative feedback between cholesterol–intake and the body's own cholesterol production in the liver plays a prominent role. The more cholesterol from the outside the less cholesterol production in the liver. Without cholesterol in your body you're dead, as most hormones have a chemical structure derived from cholesterol. Enjoy your meal, but don't start your breakfast with a 30-eggs omelette, like the former King Faroek of Egypt (1922-1965, his weight was 140 kilos in his later years).

Chapter 30

Stress and aging

Here I'll present the topic STRESS in a nutshell. For an in depth treatment of STRESS I refer the reader to my book **STRESS without STRESS** (Strengholt, 250 pp).

Chronic stress accelerates aging.
But stress is not merely a matter of circumstances, but chiefly the subjective perception. One person taking care of a demented partner or parent experiences this as chronic stress, another as feather light volunteer aid.

The Nobel prize winner Elizabeth Blackburn (see chapter 13) and the psychologist E.S. Epel etal studied the relationship between chronic stress and telomere length (a direct marker of aging) in women who had to take care of a demented family member for years and who according to a questionnaire experienced this as stressful. What was the outcome?[47] The women in this group had considerably shorter telomeres than women in the similar control group, which proves conclusively that stress accelerates the (fundamental) aging process, since, as we have seen in chapter 13, telomere length determines the biological age of the individual. To refresh your memory: telomeres are the plastic ends of a shoelace, if the latter represents a chromosome (chapter 13).

But long before the discovery of telomeres as time clock of aging this association between stress and aging had been well documented by 'aging-tests' (comparable to IQ-tests). For example a 35-year

---

47 Epel, E.S., Blackburn, E.H., et.al. *Accelerated telomere shortening in response to life stress,* Proc. Natl. Acad. Sci USA, 101, 17312, 2004.

old leading a stressful life turned out to have a 'biological age' of 55 so, greatly 'aged'.

But it is often hard to get out of a stressful life style in the case of nursing a demented family member. Only death or unbearable deterioration (admission) can bring relief.

Let me mention in passing the case of a young couple (early forties) who came to my office a long time ago. They ran a very successful business with lots of profits and a lot of stress. Because of all the stress they decided to sell the business and breed sheep instead. Little profit, but, oh, what peace and quiet ...

But not many businessmen would be willing to make such a radical switch.

Stress in a bad marriage with a cold-hearted partner is perhaps the worst form of stress, as the following passage taken from my book *Stress Without Stress* illustrates.

Professor Groen studied 10,000 employees in Israel. This study lasted 5 years. It was designed to answer the question what psychological factors were causally related to the development of angina pectoris (chest pains caused by narrowed coronary arteries). It turned out that besides the well-known risk factors for atherosclerosis chronic relation-stress played a significant role. The men who were in a bad marriage (they judged their wives as cold, indifferent and hard) and who, due to this, constantly felt tense and fatigued, turned out to have the highest risk to develop angina pectoris and sustain a heart attack.[48]

Chronic relation-stress ('bad marriage') speeds up aging and increases the risk of cardio-vascular disease. Sometimes you must stop and pause and look at your life-situation from some distance ('helicopter-thinking'). Continue, stay unhappy, age prematurely, or cut the knot? Not everyone can make a choice, even if it were only for financial reasons. It is high time for some scholar to write a doctoral thesis on 'The Economics of Love'.

---

48 Medalie, J., M.Snyder, J.J. Groen, Am. J. Med.,55, 583, 1973

What to do to slow down the accelerated aging as a result of chronic stress if it keeps you in its iron grip?

In any case you should take all measures to slow down the shortening of your telomeres, as discussed in chapter 38: fish-oil capsules, exercise, meditation, a multi-vitamin, vitamin D3, carnosine and – when possible – TA-65, the only preparation proven to extend telomeres both in test animals and in man. Are you imprisoned in the treadmill of chronic stress? Return immediately to chapter 14.

Chapter 31

Bald? A matter of choice

Getting grey is awful, but getting bald is far worse. It is the silent fear of many older men. After fifty the hair gets thinner and more and more hairs are lost. However the drug called finisteride (chemical name) prevents hair loss in most cases. How does it work?

In men a small percentage of testosterone (5 percent or less) is converted within the body into the strongly androgenic hormone dehydrotestosterone, or DHT. DHT is the real culprit, the cause of baldness in older men.

Finisteride inhibits the action of the enzyme that converts testosterone into DHT. So, no DHT is formed, no hair loss. Why is DHT so bad? Because it shrivels the hair follicle.

The branded product Propecia (finisteride 1,5 mg) has been developed against hair loss. I'm using it since 1993 and I have not lost a single hair since. As the hair is also a bit thicker it gives the impression of a thicker mop of hair. Despite the use of Propecia the quality of my hair has further deteriorated over the years to the point that I had to keep it almost as a crew-cut to prevent it from looking like 'straw in the wind'.

However, since 2010, when I started taking TA-65 to lengthen my telomeres (including those of the hair follicle cells, see chapter 13) my hair has improved enormously, allowing me to have my hair 'long' and populating some very strange balding spots with new hairs.

As TA-65 is expensive you may well lose all your hair just ordering it.

Instead of TA-65 you can use the miracle substance C60 (chapter 42) to greatly improve the growth and quality of your hair. C60 is very cheap and very effective.

A preparation similar to Propecia is Avodart, which contains the substance dutasteride that works in the same way as finisteride: by blocking the enzyme that converts part of testosterone into DHT.

Although officially banned for women because of pregnancy concerns, older women can safely use these products, as attested by Dutch dermatologists who have shown them to be effective in the majority of women with hair loss.

Surgical procedures such as hair transplantation, stem cell –techniques, etc. must be left out of consideration.

Warning
Since finisteride and dustasteride act by blocking the production of DHT that plays a significant role in libido in both men and women there is a risk that libido may be affected.

Then the choice is between baldness and sex.

A stewardess told me in my office that she lost her partner by using Avodart. She would rather lose her partner than her hair.

Chapter 32

How to protect myself against cancer

One in three gets cancer in his life, and the older you are the greater the risk.

As I mentioned before, the chance of an 80-year-old to get cancer is 2000 times greater than that of a 18-year-old. Mark you 2000 times, not 2000 percent. An enormous difference, which you fully appreciate when you compare this number with the increased risk of heavy smokers of getting lung cancer: forty times (40x) higher risk than non-smokers! If 40 times is a lot, what is 2000 times?

No-one can completely avoid the risk and it is not just a matter of age, but to a large extent a matter of life-style and eating habits.

Cancer is a tombola, but you can do much to decrease the risks.

As was already mentioned in the earliest chapters important measures are:

- eat little meat and animal fats (avoid processed meat; ham, sausage, etc.).
- eat a lot of vegetables and fruit.
- avoid sugar (and sugary drinks).
- maintain your ideal weight.
- take some exercise (3 hours walking a week).
- avoid negative stress.

These measures which I primarily recommend to greatly slow down the process of aging, also offer protection against cancer.

But don't take my word for it. These recommendations are confirmed by the **Expert Report of the World Cancer Research Fund** which was published in 2007.

The report bore the telling title **Food, Nutrition, Physical Activity and the Prevention of Cancer: a Global Perspective.**

As mentioned in Wikipedia it took six years to compile the report. Starting from 22.000 studies 7000 were selected on the basis of strict criteria. This information was analysed by an Expert Panel of 21 world-renowned scientists under the chairmanship of professor Sir Michael Marmot. The Panel made 10 recommendations, among which:

- **Body weight:** be as slim as possible within the normal range (see also chapter 6).
- **Exercise:** be physically active as part of your daily life.
- **Food and drinks that increase body weight**: Restrict the consumption of calorie-rich (high-fat) foods; avoid sugary drinks.
- **Vegetable foods**: Eat mainly food of vegetable origin.
- **Animal food**: Restrict the consumption of red meat and avoid processed meat.

Points
Studies show that people who eat little fruit and vegetables run twice the risk of getting cancer than people with a high consumption.

- Compared to the vegetables-fruit diet the meat-fat diet significantly increases the risk of skin cancer (especially the squamous form).

- Of course, as we discussed in earlier chapters, the use of cooking at high temperatures (baking, broiling, oven, etc.) should be restricted because of the formation of AGE's. AGE's promote the risk of colon cancer in particular.

- It almost goes without saying that smoking and the excessive consumption of alcohol should be avoided. Smoking not only increases the risk of lung cancer, but of many other cancers, including pancreas cancer. It is best to restrict alcohol to one glass of wine a day or its equivalent.

- Certain cancers, among which prostate cancer, are strongly associated with overweight. Overweight increases the risk of all cancers, which is connected to what professor Michael Pollak (see chapter 8) formulates: "cancer loves the metabolic environment of the obese person."

- As many people know plants in the cabbage family (cabbage, broccoli, Brussels sprouts, etc.) offer extra protection against cancer.

Drugs and supplements for cancer prevention
Prevention of course doesn't mean that you won't get cancer, but that you can lower your cancer risk, for example from 1 in 3 to 1 in 30 (3 percent chance instead of 30 percent).

In chapters 6 and 7 the significance of metformin for cancer prevention has been extensively discussed.
If you are able to obtain this drug from your doctor to slow down aging, you're at the same time strongly protected against cancer, cutting your risk in half.
Substances like selenium, curcuma (also in capsule), etc. also offer protection.
This is not the place to discuss all possibilities for protection.
I'll confine myself to a personal note; what I use daily as part of my cancer prevention program:

Metformin,
curcuma (capsule),
selenium (200 mcg),
naltrexone (1.5 mg per tablet), three tablets daily.

> The latter requires some comment.
> Naltrexone in a dosage of 100 mg is a drug against addiction that has been available since the early eighties. It had been shown that in very low dosage (3 mg daily) it

offers protection against cancer (40 percent less chance of getting cancer). The very low dosed naltrexone is referred to as LDN (Low Dose Naltrexone). Even in the case of an existing cancer LDN results in a significant percentage of cases in stabilising or shrinking the tumour (see google). But this is a different story.

LDN, low dose naltrexone, has no side effects and is available by prescription only. You may try to contact my favourite pharmacy, the Dutch pharmacy Mierlo-Hout, www.mierlohout.nl, for further information.

Important note
In chapter 42 the 'miracle drug' against aging C60 is discussed. Since it is both safe and cheap while studies have shown that it boosts the immune system in humans and greatly retards the growth and spread of human cancers implanted in test animals, it seems natural to recommend this substance for cancer prevention. Although this is an 'extrapolation' (so, not scientifically watertight) based on 'Sherlock Holmes reasoning', the following finding is a further argument for the use of C60 in cancer prevention, apart from its enormous potential for your life span (See chapter 42).

In the animal experiment discussed in chapter 42, 80 percent of the rats in the control group) died of cancer.

The rats treated with C60, who lived nota bene almost twice as long all stayed cancer-free: an astonishing result.

I'm using C60 since 2013. If you'd ask me why, I would answer: "As protection against cancer and as a putative life-extender in man". Let's drink to that!

Chapter 33

DHEA memory and Alzheimer's disease

Warning: this is the 'hardest' chapter.
According to American data half the people over 86 are demented or growing demented. Just as with rheumatoid arthritis the process is insidious, beginning with innocent lapses of short-term memory. Cortisol damage to the memory centre (hippocampus) plays a crucial role in the process. DHEA-supplementation acts protective and thus prevents dementia and memory loss.

There are many roads to Rome and DHEA (de-hydro-epi-androsterone) follows different paths to reach its goal: longer life. In this chapter I shall confine myself to one path, an important and at the same time exceptionally interesting path, or better, *'highway'*.

Just like the stress hormone cortisol (more generally it is called gluco-cortisol), DHEA is produced in the adrenal glands (adrenals). This paired endocrine gland sits atop both kidneys. Just like the sex gland and the thyroid gland the adrenal gland is under the control of the 'master gland', the pituitary, which is connected by a stalk to the underside of the brain. The pituitary gland produces for each of the above-mentioned glands a specific hormone that stimulates that gland to produce more of its own hormones.

For example, when the pituitary produces extra TSH (thyroid stimulating hormone) the thyroid will produce more thyroid hormone (thyroxin). When the pituitary produces extra LH (luteinising hormone, then – in the male - the sex gland (testis) will produce extra testosterone.

The adrenal gland is stimulated to produce more cortisol and DHEA by the pituitary hormone ACTH (adreno-cortico-trophic hormone).[49]

In all cases the pituitary hormone reaches its target organ via the bloodstream (Note: this rule holds generally: all hormones reach their target organ(s) via the bloodstream).

But just as in the case of your room thermostat and the flushing mechanism of your toilet there is (negative) feed-back at play.
Let me use a plumber's example of negative feedback.

When you have flushed your toilet the water will rise till the cistern is full. As you know there is a vertical pipe in the cistern with an opening at the top that can be closed by a valve.
 The position of the valve is regulated by a float. The more the float rises with the water level, the more the float decreases the water flow, until at the highest position of the float the flow stops completely.

The higher the production of the dependent quantity (e.g. cortisol), the more the production of the regulator (here ACTH) is checked, and conversely.

If the so-called end-organ (adrenals, testis, thyroid, etc.) is surgically removed the master gland, the pituitary, meets with no opposition and so will produce maximal amounts of the stimulating hormone in question. For example in the case of castration or after the menopause (the ovaries are 'dead') the pituitary will produce the maximal amounts of LH, which is reflected as high LH blood levels.
 If the (paired) adrenals are removed, then the brake on ACTH is lost, resulting in maximal ACTH blood levels.
 Conversely, if cortisol, or its 'cousin', 'dexamethasone', is sup-

---

[49] The meaning of this acronym is evident from the following: *Adrenals, Cortisol,* etc. are produced in the *cortex* (of the adrenals), while '*trophe*' means to stimulate. Thus, *adreno-cortico-trophic-hormone, ACTH.*

plied orally or by injection the ACTH production is greatly reduced.

The pituitary 'knows' there is enough cortisol in the blood and so the production of this hormone is cut off.

But how does the pituitary 'knows' this? In your house the thermostat is in the living room while the heater is elsewhere, in the cellar, the attic.

Where is the sensor measuring the cortisol blood level located? In the pituitary? No, the sensor is elsewhere, deep in the brain, in a region called the hippocampus.

The hippocampus is very important, for it is the seat of our short-term memory.

Parkinson and Alzheimer's disease
During aging brain cells are being lost, but in the hippocampus and in another region, the substantia nigra (black substance) it is like a battlefield, as can be seen on CT-scans (CT = 'computed tomography'). Little wonder that our memory deteriorates with aging: too many memory cells are dying off in our hippocampus.

The high 'mortality' in that other region (the substantia nigra) is the cause of another disease of aging: tremor. In the substantia nigra the substance dopamine is produced and with increasing cell death the production of dopamine dwindles (after 50) with about 12 percent per decennium. If this process accelerates Parkinson's disease occurs, as dopamine offers protection against tremor.

So, accelerated cell death in the substantia nigra results in Parkinson, while an accelerated cell death in the hippocampus (our main point of interest), leads to Alzheimer's disease.

Let me mention in passing that many Parkinson patients exhibit to a lesser-or-greater degree Alzheimer's symptoms and conversely, Alzheimer's patients often show signs of Parkinson.

Why this digression, you may wonder. Well, because after 40 cortisol and the hippocampus become entangled in a kind of vicious circle resulting in damage to hippocampus cells from 'too much' cortisol. This results in a deterioration of the functioning of the hippocampus sensor for cortisol, by which the ACTH production is insufficiently curbed. This results in a further (abnormal) increase in the cortisol production, this resulting in more damage to the sensor: in other words, the vicious circle is complete.

The result of this bizarre circle dance is that hippocampus cells die off more rapidly, which results in our memory deteriorating (too) rapidly and the risk of Alzheimer's disease looms large.

Cortisol: the death hormone
Cortisol, one of the afore-mentioned stress hormones, brings our body in supreme readiness when in danger (stress, lion).

But chronically too much cortisol – as in aging after 40 – is harmful to our health. It not only causes high blood pressure, diabetes, bone-marrow damage, stomach bleedings and many other ill-effects, but too much cortisol also accelerates the aging process because it shrinks the thymus – a central factor in aging and the 'conductor' of our immune system: thymus atrophy.

Moreover (too much) cortisol is a specific poison for the brain cells (a so-called neurotoxin) in general and for the hippocampus cells in particular.

In short, cortisol and its kind (prednisone, etc.) are very noxious substances and the asthma patient or the rheumatic patient who has to take these steroids for years is – with regard to aging – definitely not to be envied.

Let me digress a little to illustrate the toxicity of cortisol.

An extreme example of its toxicity is seen in the salmon. It swims upriver to its breeding place. Some weeks after spawning it dies. When one studies the fish at this stage it turns out that the adrenals are enormously enlarged. The fish is full of ulcers. There immune system has completely broken down, so they are also full of bacteria and parasites. No wonder the salmon dies so quickly.[50]

---

50   Robertson,O. and B.Wexler, Science,125, 1295, 1957.

But how do we know for sure cortisol is the cause of death? Simple. If after spawning the adrenals are removed they just keep on living for over a year, instead of just a few weeks.

As you can see: cortisol is the 'death-hormone', but fortunately our condition is not as bad as that of the salmon, or the marsupial mouse in Australia, where the male dies shortly after the love season.[51]

Misfortune after sex. All to do with the exile from paradise! Adam is said to have lived 930 years. We – if we're lucky - barely reach 93 years. Is our high cortisol production after puberty the cause of our early demise, just as in de salmon and the Australian mouse, only smeared out in time?

A ridiculous question, with as we shall see, a grain of truth.

The best speculative scientific answer would be: Adam produced a lot of telomerase, keeping his telomeres long (chapter 13). We have lost that capacity.

The neurotoxic action of cortisol

Right, we have seen that the cortisol receptors are located in the hippocampus, just as your thermostat is in the living room rather than near the heater. How do these hippocampus cells 'smell' the presence of cortisol in the blood? Because of the presence of so-called cortisol receptors in their cell membrane (cell skin). Cortisol fits in these receptors like a key in a lock.

Each type of hormone has its own receptors in the body. The female hormone estradiol has estradiol receptors in the uterus, the breasts, etc. That's why that in puberty the breasts enlarge, but not the stomach where the receptors are absent.

In the male in puberty the penis, where testosterone receptors are present, grows bigger, while in the nose – with the exception of that of Cyrano de Bergerac – these receptors are fortunately missing.

So, the cortisol receptors in the hippocampus that stick out like

---

51   Mc.Donald, L. et al, J. Endocrin., 108, 63, 1986.

mini-antennae to measure the cortisol blood level are the components of the hippocampus sensor.

It is clear that when the hippocampus cells die off and so disappear, the sensor becomes less sensitive for cortisol (the technical term is: glucocorticoid resistant), which results in a too weak inhibition of the ACTH production (and release). Due to this the adrenals continue to produce too much cortisol, leading to a vicious circle.

How did it start? Chicken or egg? How come the nerve cells in the hippocampus die off much more quickly even in normal healthy people than in the rest of the brain where the cell loss is small?

The answer is:
Hippocampus cells die because they have been exposed for a lifetime to the neurotoxic influence of cortisol and similar substances (gluco-corticoids derived from the adrenals).[52]

It should not come as a surprise that the gateway to this calamity are the thousands of cortisol antennae at the surface of the hippocampus cell (in the appendix of this chapter the mechanism will be further examined).

Naturally these conclusions are based on animal experiments. When you give test animals extra cortisol over an extended period (in physiological doses) it turns out that hippocampus cells degenerate or die in large numbers. Conversely, the hippocampus remains well preserved in animals in which the adrenals are for the most part removed.[53]

That this also holds in man follows from the fact that in patients with an adrenal tumour producing large quantities of cortisol (Cushing's syndrome) the CT-scan shows a considerable shrinkage (atrophy) of the hippocampus.[54]

---

52 In the case of true Alzheimer's disease (40 percent of dementia cases) the neurological degeneration is the primary factor ('plaques', 'tangles'). The 'adrenal factor' exacerbates the process via a vicious circle.
53 Landfield, P., et al, 1981 *Science*.no 214, p.581.
    Sapolsky, R., et al, 1990, *J. Neuroscience,* no. 10, p.2897.
54 Starkman, M., et al, 'Hippocampal volume, memory dysfunction and cortisol levels in patients with Cushing's syndrome, *Biol. Psychiatry,* no. 32, p. 756.

If it is true that the cortisol sensor is located in the hippocampus and that the hippocampus atrophies with aging - which results in the sensor becoming less sensitive - you may expect that with aging the cortisol level in the blood increases. In that case increase of cortisol level is a (premature) aging phenomenon, just like the gradual increase in blood pressure and cholesterol. This turns out to be the case, as has been found by the Dutch team of E. de Kloet and others.[55]

It goes without saying that chronic stress (increased cortisol) also leads to accelerated cell death in the hippocampus, resulting in a decrease in memory function.

When you compare different age groups you will find that the average blood pressure slowly rises with age. Whereas in the young this value is 120/80, it is 150/95 at 70. But of course some of the elderly may have the youthful blood pressure of 120/ 80.

This also holds for cortisol values and those who at an older age still enjoy youthful (low) cortisol values remain biologically younger and retain their youthful memory and mental capacity, one of the hall marks of 'successful aging'.

The small memory lapses occurring at middle age are a harbinger of the accelerated hippocampus shrinkage by cortisol damage.[56]

The decline in memory after 45 is 'normal'. But it is possible to inhibit this 'normal' loss of cell loss in the hippocampus in such a way that at 70 the CT-scan does not show a 20 percent loss, but only a 5 percent loss or less. This protects against Alzheimer's disease, but perhaps even more importantly your memory will remain strong en your brain sharp after 50. This can be achieved by DHEA supplementation, the subject of the next paragraph.

DHEA supplementation inhibits cortisol production.
In order to gain a good understanding of the inhibitory role of DHEA on the cortisol production – and thus on the hippocampus aging - the following observation is in order.

---

55 See van Eekelen, J., et al, 1991, *Neurobiolog. Aging,* no13, p.159.
56 Of course, a second possibility is primary death of neurons as a result of a neurological disease (Alzheimer's), local atherosclerosis (ischemia), etc.

DHEA, that - like cortisol – is formed in the adrenal gland(s) is – like cortisol – under ACTH regulation.[57]

During stress both the production of cortisol and DHEA rises under the influence of (the stimulating action) of an increased ACTH production. With aging the DHEA production in the adrenals diminishes. Since, with aging, cortisol production increases and DHEA production decreases it follows that the DHEA/cortisol quotient decreases.

As the Japanese researcher M. Namiki showed the accelerated aging by decreased DHEA production is made worse by the simultaneous decrease in the DHEA/cortisol quotient.[58]

The pituitary produces the hormone ACTH. Via the bloodstream it reaches the adrenals where it stimulates cortisol production. Without the ACTH stimulus no cortisol production. It's that simple. Cortisol is the stress hormone, so in a stress situation (a charging bull or a fight with your wife or the IRS) the cortisol production must rise to prepare the body for flight or fight. That occurs in the higher brain centres (cortex), from where *stimulatory* nerve impulses are sent to the hypothalamus, which in its turn stimulates the pituitary to discharge more ACTH into the bloodstream.

The result is that the ACTH level in the blood rises and that constitutes the stimulus for the adrenal gland to produce more cortisol.

The cortisol level should not soar. The 'brake' is in the hippocampus where the cortisol sensor is located. If it registers that the cortisol level gets too high, the hippocampus sends *inhibitory* signals to the hypothalamus, which transmits this 'inhibitory message' to the pituitary telling it to make less ACTH and thus curb the cortisol production.[59]

It is thus important to realize that during stress the ACTH production rises as a result of activating signals from the cerebral cor-

---

57 ACTH is not the only feedback regulator of DHEA. See e.g. Kreitzer P.M.,et.al. (1989) *J Clin Endorc.Metab.* No. 69, p. 1309.
58 Namiki, M. (1994). *NRIZ Journal.* No. 31, p. 85.
59 inhibitory impulses.

tex, while the feed-back regulatory mechanism insures that the cortisol production remains at the desired level by inhibitory impulses from the hippocampus.

But what happens if the cortisol production threatens to get too low? Then, obviously, the pituitary must produce more ACTH to stimulate the adrenal gland to produce more cortisol.

This happens as follows. The hippocampus sensor senses that the cortisol level in the blood tends to be low, so the hippocampus will send *fewer* inhibitory impulses. This results in an increased production of ACTH by the hypothalamus-pituitary system. The end-result is that the cortisol production increases again, thus restoring the equilibrium.

Gradual degeneration of the hypothalamus

Let us for a moment forget everything about stress. You're living on an idyllic island with nothing to worry about. What happens to your pituitary regulator under these ideal conditions?

Suppose (for the sake of an example) that the ideal cortisol value in blood (the cortisol set point) is 80.

Now it can happen that the adrenal gland – e.g. as a result of extra vitamin C or vitamin B5 - becomes too active 'on its own'. Then the cortisol level rises. This is registered by the hippocampus sensor, that decides the cortisol value is too high (at 82, say) and thus starts curbing the pituitary.

The hippocampus thus sends additional inhibitory impulses to the pituitary (via the hypothalamus) resulting in a lower cortisol production, thus restoring the equilibrium. The cortisol value drops from 82 back to 80.

But what happens in the course of aging?

The hippocampus slowly degenerates, resulting in a decline of the sensor, which becomes less sensitive, 'hard of hearing' you might say, so that the warning signal (deviation from the value of 80) needs to be greater (greater than 82) before it registers ('hears') and responds.

But his 'voice', too, becomes less loud. He can't 'shout' to the hypothalamus with the same intensity anymore, telling it to warn the pituitary to make less ACTH. When the cells in your inner ear decrease in number your sense of hearing will diminish. The signal (in this case sound) will have to be stronger before you can hear it. The same is true when the cell population of the hippocampus becomes smaller. In our example the set point is 80. An intact hippocampus responds at a deviation of 2 points (blood cortisol value 82).

The hippocampus that has become 'deaf' due to cell loss, will only respond when the deviation is greater than 2. For example when the cortisol level has risen to 90 (instead of 82), a deviation of 10 points. Clearly not a good thing, but what is worse is that the message from the hippocampus that eventually reaches the pituitary becomes *weaker.*

If for example a youthful hippocampus fires 1000 impulses per minute to instruct the pituitary to produce less ACTH, the older hippocampus (from cell loss, etc.) will only be able to fire 500 impulses. What will be the result? The pituitary will be far less curbed than is required to bring the cortisol level of 90 back to 80. So, because the ACTH production is insufficiently curbed, the end-result of this simplified (so, fictitious) example, is that the cortisol level remains too high, say, 85 instead of 80.

This will initiate a vicious circle. Too high cortisol leads to more damage, so there will be more cell loss in the hippocampus, etc.

Progressive memory loss, poor concentration, etc. are the inevitable consequences.

But the darkest hour is just before the dawn: DHEA supplementation.

Aging: simply rotten

With aging – after 35 - the production of DHEA in the adrenals decreases steeply. This is not due to a decrease in the ACTH production in the pituitary, but is simply the result of a programmed progressive exhaustion of those adrenal cells involved in the production of DHEA.

The decreased production of DHEA is unfortunate, since both, cortisol and DHEA, are regulated, via the negative feedback - discussed above – by ACTH. Since ACTH stimulates the production of cortisol and DHEA, while, conversely, these hormones curb the production of ACTH. It is obvious that if the production of DHEA *stops,* one of both brakes will fall out *completely.*

Also, it should be obvious, that even if the hippocampus is undamaged the cortisol level would be too high. For, after all, one brake has fallen out!

Instead of the desired value 80 the cortisol value would be – even when the hippocampus is intact - be too high, 84, say. Indeed, a complex situation, hard to grasp.

But with aging the DHEA production (and blood level) never drops to zero. That means that one ACTH–brake does not fall out completely, but becomes weaker.

The end-result will be the same: the cortisol level rises.

So, getting older is bad for your brain, because as a result of the vicious circle the hippocampus deteriorates further and in addition this vicious circle is strengthened by the decreased DHEA production resulting in the pituitary producing even more ACTH.[60]

The solution: DHEA supplementation

A typical 50-year-old has about a third the DHEA value of a 30-year-old (In terms of DHEA blood value, say, 2000 instead of 6000 mg/dl.).

A 90-year-old has only one-hundredth of the youth-values (60). DHEA supplementation may restore the DHEA blood level to a youthful level (6000 mg/ml) in the 50+.

This means that he high DHEA value in the blood is registered by the DHEA-sensor in the hypothalamus, by which the ACTH production is automatically curbed. Less ACTH means less cortisol (production) which is desirable. But it also means curbing the body's own production of DHEA in the adrenals and that is not a good thing, you might think.

---

60   The hormone DHEA does not influence the ACTH production via the hippocampus but directly via the hypothalamus.

Actually that's irrelevant since what matters is the blood DHEA level and whether that is maintained by the body's own production or by swallowing a pill is irrelevant.

Supplementation of DHEA to youth values, monitored by blood tests, curbs the ACTH production of the pituitary and thus (in older people) the undesirable high cortisol production in the adrenals.

The end-result is breaking the vicious circle leading to mental deterioration and, in many persons, even to severe memory loss and dementia, the result of cortisol induced degeneration of the hippocampus.

This is the crux of the matter. As a therapeutic 'complication' it should be mentioned that (as shown by computer modelling) it is desirable in older people to give more DHEA than is required to restore youthful blood DHEA-values.

In the numerical example presented above, if you bring the blood level of DHEA to 10,000 (instead of the youthful level of 6000 mg/ml.), you will achieve a 'supernormal' curbing of the ACTH production, resulting in the cortisol production staying safely low, despite the 'deaf' cortisol sensor.

DHEA supplementation extends average life expectancy. Is this partially the result of this mechanism? Sure! Alzheimer (dementia) is cause of death no 4. It is obvious that prevention of one of the most important causes of death contributes to extending the average life expectancy, or, more concretely, to improving lifespan, yours and mine.

Besides regulation of the cortisol production DHEA acts through different pathways 'brain=protective', e.g. by its role as a 'growth-factor' and a powerful antioxidant.

Are there, besides DHEA, other substances that curb ACTH production? Yes, indeed: cortisol, prednisone and other synthetic adrenal steroids, but that will get you, of course, from the frying pan into the fire.

Conclusion

The most important role of DHEA supplementation in slowing progressive loss of memory and mental deterioration goes via curbing ACTH production, breaking the vicious circle that leads to progressive degeneration of the memory centre, the hippocampus.

DHEA also has the capacity to regenerate sick nerve cells via its action as a powerful 'growth factor'.

Lowering the cortisol production to safe values with the aid of DHEA supplementation (the DHEA-hippocampus therapy) is a medical treatment involving much more costs than the usual DHEA treatment, which avoids measuring the DHEA, cortisol and ACTH levels periodically.

All you have to do – like me – is swallow a capsule of 50 mg (or 100mg) DHEA daily and unless there are side-effects like, in women; undesired hair growth (upper lips), you can safely maintain this dose without the need for expensive blood tests.

Medical Appendix

The pioneer in the field of the DHEA-hippocampus therapy is professor Robert Sapolsky of Stanford University (Cal.).

1. Chronic exposure to GC (glucocortisteroids) causes accelerated aging of the hippocampus (measured by aging–markers) while the reverse is true with low GC (e.g. surgical removal of the adrenals).[61]

2. Glucose–utilisation by the hippocampus is greatly inhibited by GC's.[62] This makes the hippocampus, in the presence of high GC's, highly vulnerable for energy crises situations like hypoglycaemia and transient ischemia (diminished blood flow).[63]

    Cell death results from lack of energy supply, followed by calcium and EAA's accumulation in the neuron. (EAA's = excitory amino acid neurotransmitters).[64]

    By means of chelation therapy (removal of intracellular calcium) neuron death can be prevented at this stage (See my book *Chelation therapy*).

3. Chronic severe stress and the use of adrenal steroids (prednisone, triamcinolone, dexamethasone, etc.) promote hippocampus degeneration and with that the decline of intellectual capacity and memory.

---

61   Meaney, M., et.al. (1988), *Science,* No. 239, p. 766. and Landfield, P., et. al. (1981*), Science,* No. 214,p. 581.
62   Kadekaro, M. et.al. (1988), *Neuro Endocr.* No.47, p. 329.
63   Sapolsky, R. (1994), Utrecht: David de Waal lezing .
64   Joels, M. & E. de Kloet, (1992), *Trends in Neuroscience.* No. 15, p.25.

Chapter 34

Growth hormone: obsolete

In 1989 the medical world was surprised by a paper written by Dr. Daniel Rudman in the leading medical journal the *New England Journal of Medicine*. In his study he gave 21 men between 60 and 80 years with low growth hormone levels and symptoms of growth hormone deficiency (diminished muscle power, fatigue, poor memory, etc.) growth hormone injections during six months. The results, both 'clinical' and quantifiable were impressive. Most men got much more energy (one man who never left his couch was repairing the roof after two months and his wife called him 'Popeye'), libido was restored, etc., while the average muscle mass increased by almost 9 percent, fat mass decreased by 14.4 percent, etc. Later these results were corroborated and extended by a study by Mark Blackman et.al. of the National Institute of Aging in collaboration with the Johns Hopkins University. Rudman's paper initiated the wide use of growth hormone as an anti-aging measure and – hopefully - life-extender.

I, too ,was enthusiastic and had used it both for myself and (selected) elderly patients for a number of years in the early nineties.

I stopped using it because 1) growth hormone does not extend the lives of test animals (in some cases it shortens it), 2) because it promotes the production of the hormone-like substance IGF-1 in the liver. IGF-1 has about the same adverse actions as (excessive) insulin. Moreover, growth hormone treatment (3 injections a week) is very expensive, in the order of € 10.000 a year.

"I just bought a bottle of growth hormone. It shrunk my wallet."

If you're willing to spend such money for 'health maintenance' it would be much better to spend it on TA-65 (telomerase activator, see chapter 14).

Originally growth hormone was only used in children. Before 1985 growth hormone was obtained from the pituitary glands of deceased people. When in 1985 this was prohibited because of the risk of a kind of mad-cow disease (Creutzfeld-Jacob disease) the medical world was at its wits end. *The darkest hour is just before the dawn.* In 1985 the synthetically produced human growth hormone Protropin became available, made by bacteria containing the human gene for growth hormone in their DNA. A few years later Nutropin was developed which is identical to the natural human growth hormone.

The main reason growth hormone fell from its pedestal is that it does not increase lifespan.

This also holds for humans, as is shown by the finding in 65 midgets in Brasil with a mutation in the HGH gene (HGH = Human Growth Hormone). Despite the fact that they did not produce growth hormone they had a normal (average) lifespan.

Further a randomised study at Stanford University, published in 2007, in 220 older individuals showed that the use of HGH as anti-aging treatment is unjustified.

HGH as anti-aging therapy cannot be recommended because of 1) the proven inefficacy, 2) the very high costs and 3) its potential disadvantages (increased IGF-1 production, see above, etc.).

Oral growth hormone products or nose–sprays advertised on the internet are pure deceit.

Chapter 35

Chelation therapy for narrowed arteries

On March 27, 2013 the results of the so-called TACT study was published in the JAMA (Journal American Medical Association) on chelation therapy for narrowed arteries. The conclusion of this large-scale-multicentre double-blind statistical study sponsored by the NIH (National Institutes of Health), that took 10-years to complete and cost over 30 million dollars, was that chelation therapy is both effective and safe.

With this the efficacy of chelation therapy has been both confirmed and scientifically established in a watertight manner by an independent body, the NIH.

Medicines, stents or chelation?
Nine out of ten cardiac patients who have been treated with chelation therapy no longer need medicines, stents or a bypass operation.

Since medicines do not cure but only alleviate symptoms and stents and bypass do not add a single day to life expectancy, while chelation therapy, by removing plaques (atherosclerosis, see chapter 17) normalizes blood flow in the coronary arteries and makes the patient symptom-free many cardiac patients (including doctors) opt for chelation therapy, a treatment that cures the patient by restoring blood flow rather than simply suppressing symptoms.

If you suffer from poor circulation due to narrowed arteries as a result of atherosclerosis (heart, legs, carotid arteries, etc.) then this treatment may be of the greatest value to your health. By the way, many Europeans (from Norway, etc.) go to the USA for chelation treatment, where over 100,000 patients are treated yearly.

Read and you will be amazed.

> Chelation therapy involves the infusion of the 3 gram EDTA dissolved in 500 cc water. EDTA (ethelene–diamine-tetra-acetic acid) is a 'non-toxic' molecule that contains four acetic acid molecules as 'sub-units'. Its action is complex but in layman's terms it works just like acetic acid removing calcium from your coffee machine. As mentioned in chapter 17 and elsewhere, most people die from the complications of atherosclerosis (cardiac infarction, stroke, etc.). Chelation cleans up the arteries and is widely used both as 'prevention' and therapy. I'm a living example of 'prevention'.
>
> Since 1982, although symptom-free, I have taken over 300 EDTA infusions to keep my arteries clean, since without atherosclerosis you'll get no heart attacks and strokes (see chapter 16) the major causes of death and disability. Remember, just as your coffee machine, even after cleaning the process of clogging continues slowly over time.
>
> The calcium bound to EDTA is removed via the kidneys. According to toxicological data EDTA is safer than aspirin.
>
> EDTA = Ethylene-Diamino-Tetra-Acetic acid (tetra=four)

Historical background

Chelation therapy, administering EDTA intravenously to improve circulation by removing plaques (atherosclerosis) was developed in de late fifties by American cardiologists, among whom the Nestor professor Norman Clark. The excellent clinical results (success percentage over 90 percent) were published in leading medical journals, among which The American Heart Journal. The treatment obtained FDA approval and was widely used in the late fifties and the early sixties. Over 60 years later (2014) chelation therapy is still the most effective and safest treatment for cardio-vascular diseases due to arterial narrowing on the basis of atherosclerosis.

It is equally effective in the treatment of *claudicatio intermittens* (poor circulation in legs), narrowing of the carotid arteries and poor circulation in the brain (dizziness, etc.).

American statistical studies have shown that chelation therapy renders bypass and stents superfluous in 80 percent of the cases. In the early sixties a vicious reaction against this 'miracle cure' took place. The therapy was simple and could be applied by any GP. Too simple?

Indeed. Cardiologists and cardiac surgeons considered this a grave threat to their status and income. If family doctors would apply it on a large scale more than half their income would be lost, as anyone can deduce from the statistics. As a young Dutch doctor I happened to be at Harvard Medical School as a 'senior NIH investigator', where I worked closely with cardiologists at the Brigham's Hospital. At the time I was head of the THORAX laboratory at the University Hospital in Groningen (the Netherlands), where I was often present during heart operations for technical matters. So, I was familiar with the world of cardiologists and cardiac surgeons. Their conversations expressed great concern about the effectiveness, coupled to safety and simplicity of chelation therapy. The large-scale application of this FDA sanctioned method would be 'life-threatening' for cardiology and cardiac surgery as bypass would become a secondary choice in those cases (10 percent) where chelation was ineffective.

Though it sounds incredible, it is an iron law in organised medicine that an unwelcome treatment, whatever its merits, quickly disappears from the medical landscape if financial interests are at stake.

Within a few years chelation therapy had been discredited and forgotten despite the fact that it had been peer-reviewed in the leading medical journals and had been endorsed by the FDA (Food and Drugs Administration), known for its stringent criteria. The scandalous facts of this historical development – in which bribery of leading researches by Blue Cross to 'recant' played a crucial role - are presented in Morton Walker's classic book *The Chelation Answer,* a must for the serious reader.

Alternative or regular?

In its **origin** chelation therapy is a 'regular' treatment, developed by 'regular' doctors (cardiologists and internists) and published in leading medical journals, as mentioned earlier.

Because of the fact that it has fallen out of favour for purely 'political reasons' it is currently an alternative treatment not covered by medical insurance.

Chelate first, operate later

As the Dutch 'maverick' cardiac surgeon Dr. Peter van der Schaar states, strict medical logic dictates that the cardiac patient – except in rare cases - should be treated first with chelation therapy. Only those cases in which chelation therapy is ineffective (10 percent) qualify for bypass surgery or a stent.

Since, as official statistics show, bypass or stent do not add a single day to life expectancy and the risks compared to the absolutely safe chelation therapy are enormous, the choice of the (well-informed) patient to first go to a chelation doctor is fully rational.

Success percentages: statistical studies
The first statistical findings about the effectiveness of chelation therapy were published in 1960 in the authoritative medical journal the *American Journal of Cardiology*. The editorial stated that chelation therapy was effective in 90 percent of cases with narrowing of the legs' arteries and in 85 percent of coronary cases (N.E. Clarke, *Am.J.Cardiol.*6, 233, 1960).

Since then these findings have been confirmed by scores of studies all over the world.

When patients tell their story
Statistics are essential, but no less important for a patient considering chelation therapy are the experiences of chelation patients, the testimony of the individual. Since the sixties more than a hundred thousand cases have been documented (see e.g. Morton Walker's book *The Chelation Answer*). But since you – as it behoves - have a healthy degree of scepticism when faced with a totally unfamiliar form of treatment it seemed like a good idea to present the reports of some patients interviewed by the highly respected presenter of the long-running Dutch television program 'Around Ten', Henk Mochel.

The following text is taken from the official written report of the program on chelation therapy in 1987. So long ago? Isn't it old hat? Well, to start with: chelation is like aspirin, it never goes out of date. The findings from 1964 are the same as those in 2014. In the Netherlands chelation therapy has been the subject of a number of television programs, but what makes the 1987 program absolutely unique is that all three groups – chelation doctors, cardiologists and chelation patients - were represented in a single broadcast.

A very important point is that the program maker and presenter Henk Mochel had immersed himself in the subject and had interviewed both doctors and patients in the preparatory period. The booklet mentioned above had been written by the presenter Henk Mochel in which he documents his experiences with patients *before* the broadcast.

Here is Henk Mochel's story about his experiences with patients in the preparatory phase. It is of 'double interest' because it shows that even the sickest heart patients can be cured by chelation therapy.

Enthusiastic patients
Programs of 'Around Ten' usually have a run-up of three to four weeks. During that time we have conversations with as many persons involved as possible. Exploratory meetings with scores of patients and family and friends offer us the personal experiences with the therapy. What was most striking in these meetings was the often emotional involvement of some patients. It sometimes happened that one of the participants became so overwhelmed by emotion that he or she had to break off the story and that the partner had to take over. That happened to the 57-year-old Willy D. from Monnickendam (a village). She got her first heart attack when she was 34, a year later her second. After that she had been doing rather well for fifteen years. Till 1979. Then one day in July she was admitted to the hospital for an emergency-operation. A cardiac valve had to be replaced and two bypasses would be placed. The operation would be done in one go. This was really very dangerous, but there was no choice.

"The operation worked for a short time. Before the end of the year the symptoms returned. At first I didn't want to believe it. I thought it may be from that tube they put in your throat for insufflation. But when I put a tablet under my tongue the pain subsided and for me that was the sign that the operation had not been successful. A second operation appeared inevitable. They said: the chances that you'll make it are less than that you won't. But that very difficult second operation didn't help me one bit. Immediately after, when I was still in the hospital, the symptoms returned. During a big heart congress in the RAI [congress centre in Amsterdam] where my case was presented to a team of doctors a professor told me that they might be able to help me in his hospital. I grabbed the chance with both hands. But even catheterisation proved impossible – that became torture. So operation was out of the question. They said I had only six months to live …, and then you start searching … (Here her husband had to take over).

In one of the popular magazines we read an article about chelation therapy. Via Dr. Defares we ended up in Dr. van der Schaar's private clinic. He wanted to explore the possibility of a third operation. He took me to Houston [Texas], but there too they didn't dare to take the risk of a third operation. The only option that remained was chelation therapy."

Where major operations were unsuccessful the simple chelation treatment proved effective.

'Already after my fifth treatment [infusion] I no longer woke up at night from pain. The following morning I knew: this works. After each next treatment I felt that I was on the mend. I started to enjoy life again.'

For a long time I had been unable to read a paper or watch television because the brain vessels too didn't function normally. But because of the chelation series this too became possible. Now I'm even so strong that I can go shopping for three hours. By that time my husband is tired and wants to go home but I'm still brimming with energy. I have come back to life and that is a wonderful feeling.

Almost six years ago she was given up – she had only six months to live, the surgeons said. Now she is a healthy woman full of vitality. Once every five weeks she goes to the van der Schaar clinic for a chelation infusion [this is required in very severe cases, J.G.D.] 'I know I'll have to do it till I die, But I don't mind doing it,' she says gratefully.

Heart specialists and vascular surgeons in general are opposed to chelation therapy. It seems they also don't like to compromise themselves vis à vis their colleagues by admitting that – where their treatment failed - chelation therapy was obviously successful. For this was for instance the case with mrs. J.B.W.K-P from Mijnsheerenland [a village]. First her own story:

'Before I went to Doctor Kunst in Arkel in January 1982 I had been suffering from cardiac pains for about eight to ten years. After a thorough examination in the hospital I was told that it was angina pectoris [due to narrowed coronary vessels, J. G. D.]. Because the medicines I received didn't work, they performed a heart catheterisation which showed, the cardiologist told us, that *nothing could be done anymore*. Then I went to Dr. Kunst. I was very ill. But after four or five treatments I said to my husband: how odd, I feel very much less tired. And after a few more treatments: I believe I don't need my medicines any longer. In consultation with doctor Kunst I started to use less and less medicines and when I stopped using them I felt like being reborn, active and perfectly healthy. The doctor advised me to take another course of 20 infusions because I had been so ill. So I had had a total of forty infusions and after that I felt like a twenty-odd young woman. I was able to take on the whole world.

One of my many hobby's is pottery, which I always do in the attic. Before the chelation I couldn't climb the steep stairs, but after I tore up the stairs. In summer I go sailing and swimming as before, and walk for hours - I was just brand-new. This is six years ago and I still feel in great shape. This year we went to Portugal, then to Germany and have travelled through France with a camper."

We were curious about the reaction of the cardiologist who had told Mrs. K in 1981 that he couldn't do anything for her anymore. After the chelation treatment she had visited him once. By telephone he said he couldn't remember the case of Mrs. K anymore. That was too long ago. We could call him back in three months, perhaps he would have found her case history by then.

Fortunately we had at our disposal for the purpose of our television program the correspondence between him and the family doctor, and later, the chelation doctor, doctor Kunst. Here are some passages from the various letters (names omitted for obvious reasons).

First some passages from the letter to the family doctor of Mrs. K.-P.

Dear colleague,

On 17-8-81 your patient J.BW. K.-P., born :25-2-18 and residing in Mijnsheerenland, was admitted to our division for heart catheterisation.
Case history: Patient has angina pectoris, for which she had been treated in our outpatient's clinic for a number of years. After an initially symptom-free period the symptoms have increased in severity since the end of last year.
Patient complains of tightening pains in the middle of the chest with moderate and sometimes light physical exercise. She even gets chest pain when undressing or taking a shower with radiation of the pain to her throat. The frequency of the pain is at least once a day. She is unable to ride a bike and shopping or household work elicits chest pains. Never pain at rest or during sleep. Occasionally she uses nitro-glycerine with good results. Despite selokene, cedocard and adalat the symptoms remain.

Conclusion: 63 year-old woman with clear-cut angina pectoris symptoms. Fitness: class 2 to 3 according to NYHA [severe, J.G.D.]. Since October the symptoms have seriously worsened. Shopping, running the housekeeping, and other light physical activities are difficult. Patient even gets angina pains while undressing or taking a shower. Cold and wind are also inducing factors.
Ergometry: highly suggestive of coronary insufficiency.
Catheterisation: Serious coronary atherosclerosis [technical details omitted, J.G.D.]. Bypass-operation is being considered.

As mentioned above an operation proved to be impossible – her condition was too poor. The conclusion of the catheterisation report was: serious coronary atherosclerosis. Stenosis [narrowing] in several places of more than 50 percent and at some locations of 90 percent. After that Mrs. K.-P. visited the chelation doctor, doctor Kunst. Her cardiologist sent Kunst at his request the following letter after having examined her following chelation.

Dear colleague,

Mrs. J.B.W. K-P, born 2-5- 1918, visited on 3-24-82 the cardiology outpatient clinic.
  Case history: patient has angina pectoris, due to coronary insufficiency, as confirmed by coronary angiography. Medicinal treatment with little effect on the symptoms, but after EDTA-infusions patient is completely symptom-free.
  Medication: apart from EDTA –infusions, none.

ECG: regular sinus rhythm, normal conduction times, flat ST-segments agreeing with coronary insufficiency.

Conclusion: the condition is subjectively clearly much improved. The patient has been discharged from further policlinic check-up.

Sincerely

Cardiologist

The cardiologist told us he could not recall this case. This seems most peculiar. After all it doesn't happen every day that a cardiologist has to admit to an alternative doctor that his treatment produced a clearly observable superior result than his own.

Chelation therapy as the last straw for a patient that has been given up or is seriously ill – the opponents will say that it works on the mind rather than the body. What does it matter if you're in such a poor shape like the 53–years old Kees V. ten years ago. His story too is illustrative of the *arrogance* of some specialists.

Kees got his first heart attack in 1975 when he was 39 years old. That turned out rather well for a while, but gradually the pain returned. Kees owned his own business and had a young family and worried about the future. When he couldn't walk more than sixty yards he asked his cardiologist to examine him properly. It took four weeks before he learned the result of the examination! The doctor had a long story using fancy terms Kees didn't understand. What does it boil down to, he asked, what's the matter with me? Am I a hopeless case? Yes, the doctor said, that's what I was trying to convey. It turned out that the results of the catheterisation report had been sent to various heart centres in Europe, but in none of these places they saw a possibility for treatment.

Then I go to America, Kees said. The cardiologist, a bit annoyed, then said, 'You don't think, do you, that they know any better?' But he was determined to fight for his life. Thanks to the intervention of Dr. van der Schaar, Kees would be operated in Houston by the well-known cardiac surgeon Dr. Cooley. It was a close shave. Dr. Cooley had Kees sign a statement that he agreed to the enormous risk of the operation. Dr. Cooley put two tablets on his night table: a sleeping pill and a painkiller. Later it turned out that if Kees had taken one of these tablets the operation would have been cancelled, as his condition would not have been good enough. Seven days later Kees, who couldn't walk more than 50 meters at home, walked around the whole hospital. On the way home he carried his own suitcases to and from the airfield. Afterwards, too, he was in such good shape that he was allowed to stop taking his medicines and start working again.

But after a vacation *in the same year*, the symptoms recurred. Again a stay in the hospital, returning home after three weeks. But he could hardly walk anymore and work was out of the question. He couldn't get any further than his chair in the living room. Again he contacted Dr. van der Schaar who immediately put him on chelation therapy. The first 25 treatments twice a week and after twice a month. "I've had 54 treatments by now and I feel in optimal condition. I jog, play ice hockey, I can do everything. I just feel great! Six months after he had forbidden me to work I went back to my cardiologist. *He was baffled.* 'So, you see how a human body may recover spontaneously.' I had not been able to convince him that I owe my cure entirely to the wholesome effect of chelation therapy." [author's comment: of course he knew, but he would never admit it.]

Final note
This ends the quote from the written testimony of Henk Mochel, presenter of the weekly program "Around Ten" in the Netherlands, a critical and independent observer.

Note that when a treatment works in desperate cases such as presented above it is surely effective in 'normal cases', as established by statistics which shows that chelation is effective in 90 percent of the patients.

If you suffer from narrowed arteries (insufficient blood supply) to the heart, legs, brain, etc. you should first consider chelation therapy as your best option for a safe and permanent cure.

There are a number of excellent books on chelation therapy in English, including The Chelation Way by Dr. Morton Walker, an independent medical writer and physician, and Bypassing bypass surgery by Dr. Elmer Cranton a Harvard–trained doctor. These books are available at Amazon.

Chapter 36

Osteoarthritis (prevention) and glucosamine

Glucosamine – a substance from the exo-skeleton of crustaceans - in a dosage of 1500-3000 mg/day lessens the pain and stiffness of osteoarthritis (joint wear from loss of cartilage) and prevents osteoarthritis by the synthesis of cartilage.

I do not suffer from osteoarthritis but have been taking glucosamine for donkey's years to keep the cartilage (knee, hip) in optimum condition.

As a doctor you have at least one case printed in your memory. One of my (preventive) patients, a perfectly healthy retired businessman, used to play Jazz on the piano as a hobby. At a certain stage he had to stop because of stiff, painful fingers. He was about to sell his grand piano. I advised him to use glucosamine. After two months he was symptom-free and the white grand piano is still standing.

Glucosamine is also effective in animal models of osteoarthritis. Although the first papers on the effectiveness of glucosamine in osteoarthritis date as far back as 1970, the landmark paper appeared in the leading medical journal *The Lancet* in 2001. Since then the medical community, too, is convinced of the efficacy of this natural substance in osteoarthritis and in slowing down wear and tear.

Under the title *'Long term effects of glucosamine sulphate on osteoarthritis progression: a randomised, placebo-controlled clinical trial'* the study showed that osteoarthritis patients who had been receiving glucosamine (1500mg/day) for 3 years had no loss of cartilage in contrast to the placebo group. The cartilage loss was measured as narrowing of the synovial cleft which was 0.3 mm in the placebo group and 0.0 mm in the glucosamine group, so, no loss of cartilage.

Also, the symptoms had greatly improved in the glucosamine group, but for our purpose the preservation of cartilage is the most important.

Osteoarthritis is nothing but the loss of cartilage, the cushion that ensures that the bones do not slide against each other. At an advanced stage the cartilage is gone, so the bones slide against each other, which causes pain when moving. The redness, swelling (*hydrops*, fluid retention) are late effects, an inflammation reaction to the disastrous condition of the joint.

At 60+ almost everyone has a certain degree of cartilage loss, although most are symptom-free.

What are the symptoms? Stiffness, especially in the morning, and after sitting a long time (restaurant). At a later stage pain during movement, creaking joints and impaired movement of the joint. As mentioned redness and swelling (knee, fingers) constitute an advanced stage. The standard treatment for the pain is paracetamol and, if insufficient, ibuprofen or diclofenac. The final solution – no more pain and restriction of movement - is an operation: a new knee or new hip. Incidentally, patients using glucosamine are less likely to need an operation. For example, a three-year study of patients who had been using glucosamine for years, showed that they require significantly fewer operations than those in the control group.[65]

The Lancet paper mentioned above and other studies show that the use of glucosamine also results in a substantial reduction in the use of painkillers.

Glucosamine is a simple molecule derived from glucose and constitutes the main building block for the macromolecules of cartilage. Both *in vitro* as in test animals glucosamine normalizes (abnormal) cartilage metabolism, restores damaged cartilage and reduces local inflammation.

It is important to know that cartilage cells have the ability to produce glucosamine. This is derived from fructose with the aid

---

65   Bruyere, O, et.al. Osteoarthritis Cartilage, 16, 254, 2008.

of the enzyme (don't be alarmed) glucosamine synthetase. With advancing age the activity of this enzyme decreases resulting in a decreased production of the building block of cartilage fibres (macro-molecules). The result: narrowing and weakening of the cartilage cushion ('wear').

By glucosamine supplementation this shortage is supplemented, allowing the cartilage cells to optimally produce the cartilage fibres, i.e. cartilage. Numerous studies since 2001 have confirmed the pioneering Lancet study. Let me mention only the 2003 article in the leading journal *Archives of Internal Medicine,* entitled, *Structural and Symptomatic Efficiency of Glucosamine and Chondroitin in Knee Osteoarthritis* (*Arch. Int. Med. 163, 1514, 2003*) in which (quote), 'the highly significant efficacy of glucosamine' is shown. Of course glucosamine will not produce a cure in advanced stages of the disease.'

Chapter 37

The libido pill

Sadly the remedies for enhancing libido (sexual desire) are very limited.

The factors that weaken libido are almost unlimited. Stress is one factor. Any stewardess will tell you that the libido of the captain of a jumbo jet will be still simmering weeks after a near-crash. Drugs, from anti-hypertension pills to antidepressants, can suppress libido, while statins can affect the pleasure of orgasm in the male. But enough about the male. Only testosterone and HCG injections - which enhance the body's own testosterone production - are able to significantly increase the libido in the male, apart from fantasy and a nude beauty. Men have Viagra (which, by the way, doesn't work in the absence of sexual desire), the poor woman has nothing, although the pharmaceutical industry is frenetically searching for the 'viagra' for women. But let's get down to business. What follows refers to the problem of women: how to strengthen the libido of women.

The short answer is: with testosterone or estrogen (estradiol).

Let me begin with two anecdotes to illustrate the point as a 'blow-up'.

An Egyptian doctor told me that wealthy married men in Cairo often keep a mistress, a pretty girl from the slums, they put up in an apartment ('love-nest') for sex. They inject the poor girl with testosterone (Sustanon from Organon, the Dutch pharmaceutical company) to increase her libido. After a year or so, these girls, super-horny, start to become ugly, balding, masculinized caricatures, and are replaced by the next victim. Testosterone works wonders indeed!

The next anecdote is more personal. I was 33 and we lived in a modest street, where everyone knew each other. Auntie Jo - everybody called her so - was 81 and married to a retired 'calculator' of the famous observatory in Leyden (82).

Both were really 'old'. I'm currently 87, but compared to them I'm a teenager!

For some reason I prescribed her oestrogen (Premarin). After some weeks, she told me, her libido had reawakened to the point that one night she asked her husband in a small voice, "Jan, please come, I have become a young girl again." Jan stayed in his own bed muttering, "No, I'm not coming I'm still an old geezer."

Both cases illustrate the influence of these hormones on the libido of the female.

But before continuing, let's answer this question, "What is the most important cause of frigidity (lack of libido) in young women, apart from stress and 'boredom' in a long relationship?" **The birth-control pill**. This can be explained biologically: the woman on the pill is, hormonally speaking, in the menopause, since the pill virtually stops the production of oestrogen and testosterone in the ovaries (chapter 21). The testosterone production in the female is less than one-seventh of that in the male, but plays an important role in libido. It is true that the pill contains oestrogen (ethinylestradiol), but only in a very low dose (because of the risk of thrombosis) while this synthetic hormone is biologically of poor quality.

Moreover the pill acts on the hypothalamus (area in the brain) where the sex centre (libido) is located.

I won't bother you with tedious statistics, but add a third characteristic anecdote. In 1997 at the height of the PILL CONTROVERSY (see chapter 21) in which I was closely involved, a teacher at a girls' high school showed me a long, humorous an intelligent satirical poem composed by some of his pupils. It dealt with The Pill and all the obstacles a teenager had to overcome to finally obtain it.

The ending was: the girl did get the pill but it was no longer needed since it took away her desire (libido).

Even very young girls apparently know from their own experience what it does to your libido!

From the extensive documentation about loss of libido by the pill I quote at random from www.timelessbeauty.nl/nodesireforsex

The birth-control pill
Less desire for making love is a possible side effect of all birth-control pills. Loss of libido can also be an insidious side-effect of the Pill, Dr. Rob Beerhuizen, gynaecologist and director of the Dutch Birth Control Foundation states.

Main cause: less own testosterone
A study published in the *Journal of Sexual Medicine* in 2006 showed that birth-control pills sharply lower the testosterone content in the blood of women. As I mentioned, this hormone is largely responsible for libido and optimum sexual functioning in the female. This low testosterone results in decreased sexual interest, sexual excitement and sense of pleasure.

> Moreover the study showed that the Pill causes a sharp increase in the production of the sex hormone binding protein SHBG (*sex hormone binding globulin*), produced in the liver. The higher the SHBG content the more sex hormones are bound to the protein and the less 'free' testosterone is available for the biological actions on the tissues and organs. In this study of the action of the Pill on testosterone the researchers found that the SHBG-levels in Pill-users were four times higher than in women who had never used the Pill. This means, that even if the Pill-woman still produces (somewhere in the body) testosterone, it will not be available for normal use, like stimulating desire. Even more worrisome is that even six months after stopping the Pill (when the study was ended), the SHBG values remained elevated. No-one knows for how long, but the investigators fear that long-time exposure to the synthetic hormones in the Pill lead – via gene-activation – to a permanent gene–expression for GHBG in the liver (that is, the liver will permanently overproduce SHBG) in some women who have used the Pill, so, to permanent frigidity.
>
> Dr. Claudia Panzer, endocrinologist and author of the above-mentioned paper, stated in a press release (2006): "It is important for physicians prescribing oral contraceptives to point out to their patients potential sexual side effects, such as decreased sexual desire and arousal, decreased lubrication, and also sexual pain."
>
> Does your family doctor or gynaecologist tell you about this? Forget it!
> "*It's all in your head, ma'am.*"
> Doctors! The greatest blessing and the greatest curse …

This was the negative side, lowering desire.

What is the positive side? Can the libido in women be increased by a drug? Yes, as the anecdotes illustrate, natural oestrogen (estradiol) and testosterone may be effective, though definitely not always.

Testosterone, of course, in a low, 'physiological dose'.

The woman is sexually most in the mood for sex during ovulation (mid-cycle). Then both the estradiol production as well as the testosterone production are at their peak. Testosterone, the most powerful of the 'male' hormones that the woman produces, plays, in connection with estradiol, a defining role in the sexuality of the female. But the woman is a far more complex being than the male: mood, energy level, and wellbeing play a greater role than in men. Low testosterone production leads to fatigue and low spirits and conversely. Testosterone (administration) thus improves the sex-experience partially by more energy and better mood.

But what is too low for testosterone? While in men the 'normal' testosterone content is between 300 and 1200 ng/dl (nanogram per decilitre), the normal value in women is between 30 and 100 ng/dl. Values lower than 30 indicate a lack of testosterone. Dr. Stephen Holzapfel, director of the Sexual Medicine Counselling Unit at Women's College Hospital in Toronto states that the administration of testosterone in women with a low testosterone production (quote), "not only increases the desire for sex, but also the excitement, sense of pleasure, the lubrication and the orgasm."

Testosterone containing preparations
Although according to estimates 35-45 percent of women suffers from symptoms of low libido and the race for a 'viagra' for women is on, currently only two testosterone preparations have been specifically developed for women, viz. Intrinsa (plaster) of Proctor and Gamble and Libigel of Biosante. In many countries (including the Netherlands) these medicines are not available.

Although there are many androgens (male hormones), varying from testosterone to DHEA (dehydro-epi-andtrosterone) and androstenedione, etc. the positive effect on the sexuality of women has been firmly established only for testosterone.

In general doctors are reluctant to prescribe testosterone for women. Rightly so, since this requires expertise (interpretation of blood tests, etc.), while excess of androgens may cause irreversible changes (voice, loss of hair, clitoris enlargement, etc.).

Some progressive doctors prescribe preparations intended for men, like the gels Andorgel and Testim in low dose for women (for example Testim not daily, but one tube divided over a week or two weeks).

In Europe the European commission had granted permission for a testosterone plaster specially developed for women, Intrinsa, but in 2012 it was suspended because the vast majority of women used it 'off-label', a ridiculous bureaucratic argument.

In those countries where Intrinsa, etc. are not available the only recourse for the woman is to persuade her doctor to prescribe the gel Testim or Androgel for use divided over one week or longer rather than one a day (see above).

If the lion's skin cannot, the fox shall. Better a lie that heals … If your male partner is willing to tell his physician he is suffering from impotence, the doctor will probably prescribe Androgel or Testim, a gel which can easily be applied to a woman's skin in small doses.

Warning: never use an androgen when there is risk of pregnancy, since it adversely affects the foetus.

The lust pill is coming
The darkest hour is just before the dawn.

On May 26, 2013 an article appeared in the New York Times Magazine under the heading. **"Unexcited? There may be a pill for that."**

In the book of the well-known American medical journalist Daniel Bergner entitled *What do women want? Adventures in the Science of Female* (2013) a great deal of space is devoted to the 'lust pill', based on Lybrido based on 30 hours talks with its inventor the Dutch psychopharmacist Adrian Tuiten, proprietor of the company Emotional Brain.

A 2013 report in the leading Dutch newspaper NRC says:

"Tuiten intends to market his pill in the USA and has advanced to stage 2 trial to obtain FDA certification, which has cost 30 million dollars thus far. The funds for the next trial are already available. Tuiten showed me everything. The scans of 'lambic areas' in the brain. A FDA approved histogram, titled, "Satisfactory Sexual Events", relating to the proven effect of 'a little peak of testosterone' and a substance contained in Viagra.

All very mysterious and in comprehensible. So a brief explanation is in order.

Here the duo testosterone and the Viagra–compound acts primarily on two so-called neurotransmitters (substances secreted by neurons to communicate with other brain cells). These are dopamine and serotonine, that, just like the extensor muscles and flexors of the thigh must be 'in equilibrium'. Lybrido temporarily disrupts this equilibrium in the brain because testosterone stimulates dopamine (the lust-substance) more strongly than the Viagra-component stimulates serotonine. All very complicated, but the end-result is that via activation of certain brain areas ('limbic-system') the psyche is directly influenced: more desire for sex! Lybrido has not been developed for a better orgasm but to solve the matter of 'little desire', the problem of some 40 percent of married women. Boredom, bah, twice a week with the same too familiar partner.

The following is a quote from the above-mentioned NYT's article:

"Tuitens' pill acts differently from earlier medicines. Lybrido contains two active compounds, exquisitely timed to make their actions converge. Each substance fiddles with the interaction between serotonine and dopamine in such a way that serotonine dominates."

But enough biochemistry!
Lybrido has a coating with a peppermint taste that melts in the mouth. When the coating is gone the woman swallows the rest

of the tablet which contains "Viagra" with 'slow-release'. "Viagra" induces, together with testosterone, an increased blood flow in the genitals resulting in increased sensitivity of the lust-nerve endings. Together they also stimulate the mind to be more conscious of erotic stimuli and both help to stimulate the dopamine networks in the brain. Result: increased libido, more desire.

This is the theory. How about its implementation.

Bergner (see above) interviewed a number of test persons (married women in a longlasting relationship), who were involved in a double-blind study of Librido. I quote from the NYT's article:

"We had sex five times a week and before only once a week", Zita told me, shortly after she had used up her supply of Lybrido. "With Lybrido", she said, "I wanted sex, even after sex. I stayed horny, so I stayed awake at night. I just wanted more." When I asked what her husband thought about the use of that medication, she laughed. "Happy," she said.

According to all indications Lybrido will be available in the USA, after FDA endorsement, in 2016. Husbands, stock up on Viagra!

Chapter 38

Supplements against telomere shrinkage

As we have seen in chapters 13 and 14 telomere lengthening means cell rejuvenation while curbing telomere shortening results in slowing down the aging of the cell and postponement of cell death. We are as old or as young as our cells, the unit of life.

Currently the only proven way to lengthen telomeres is by means of the expensive TA-65 (chapter 14). Can we slow down the rate of telomere shrinkage and so keep the cell 'youthful' longer? An important question for those who do not use TA-65, but also for those who do? For, after all, without slowing the time-dependent telomere shortening the use of TA-65 is like filling the bath with the drain wide open.

Our telomeres get shorter, the drain is wide open. The question arises: can we reduce the drainage, inhibit the rate of shortening of our telomeres?

Each year our telomeres shorten by 40-100 base pairs (don't be alarmed, see chapter 13). The greatest part of the shortening is not due to cell division, but to the damage by free radicals (inflammation, see chapter 13).

Here I'm simply going to tell you what supplements to take to curb this shortening and thus to maintain the youthful condition of your cells longer.

The data are taken from the authoritative book **The Immortality Edge** by the telomere experts Michael Fossel, Greta Blackburn and Dave Woynarowski published by Wiley in 2011.

I shall not bother you with extensive references, but only mention one scientific study with each supplement.

Here we go.

Telomere shortening is inhibited by the following supplements:

1. multi-vitamin preparation
2. omega-3 fish oil
3. vitamin D3
4. carnosine

ad 1) A high-dosed multi-vitamin preparation (see chapter 25) slows down telomere shortening, as is shown in Q. Xu's paper entitled *Multivitamin Use and Telomerase Length in Women*, that appeared in the American Journal of Clinical Nutrition, 89, 1857, 2009.

ad 2) Omega-3 fishoil capsules are – in sufficient amounts - effective against telomere shortening. What is the effective dose? The active components are EPA and DHA. The total dose – EPA+ DHA - should be 100mg or more a day. The braking action of fish oil on telomere shortening has been demonstrated for instance by the study of R. Farzaneh-Far et.al. entitled *Association of Marine Omega-3 Fatty Acid Levels with Telomere Aging in Patients with Coronary Heart Disease,* that appeared in the Journal of the American Medical Association (JAMA, 33, 250, 2010). Those who had the highest consumption of omega-3 via food had the longest telomeres and vice versa. This is possibly the most important supplement to keep your telomeres in shape.

ad 3) A large study of female twins in England that compared telomere length with vitamin D content found that women with higher vitamin D values had longer telomeres. The difference between those with the highest concentrations and those with the lowest was the equivalent of five years telomere aging. The action of vitamin D is probably the slowing down of inflammation (free radicals). For biochemical reasons it is best to use vitamin D3 (cholecalciferol), at a dose of 3000 IU daily (between 2000-5000 IU).

ad 4) Carnosine, a natural substance in meat (carne=meat, so, also in your own body, slows down the shortening of telomeres, as has been established *in vitro* (Petri-dish).

The study appeared in *Biochemical and Biophysical Research Communications,* 324, 911, 2004.

The recommended dosage is 500 mg a day or higher. If you eat a lot of meat you will get a lot of carnosine daily. Vegetarians who wish to conserve their telomeres should definitely use a L-carnosine supplement.

Of course the above-mentioned four supplements offer many more benefits than discussed here. For example, a low vitamin D content is associated with increased mortality (S.B. Kritschevsky et.al. *Journal of Clinical Endocrinology & Metabolism* ,31, 1551, 2012), while low vitamin D values are also associated with most diseases of aging, from heart disease to cancer. In part these effects may be ascribed to the protective effect of vitamin D on telomere length. Within 'normal limits' this holds: the higher your vitamin D content the better you're protected against old age diseases and premature death.

Carnosine offers many benefits: for example it is a powerful antioxidant and (in test animals) it extends life expectancy (Example: mice treated with carnosine have twice the chance of reaching maximal lifespan (of the species) than untreated mice).

Carnosine offers a powerful protection against glycation and thus protects against cataract, neuropathy, etc. (for glycation see chapter 23).

Summary

You can slow down the 'natural' telomere shortening by the following food supplements:

1. orthomolecular (high-dose) multi-vitamin
2. omega-3 fish-oil (EPA+DHA 1000mg or more)
3. vitamin D3 (2000-5000 IU/day)
4. carnosine (500-1000 mg/day)

Since the length of your telomeres determines the 'age' of your cells and we are as old as our cells, you slow down by means of these supplements the aging process at a fundamental level. For, aging is determined by the time clock in the cell, the telomere (chapter 13). Indeed, with these 4 supplements you slow down the aging process.

With the aid of the telomerase activator TA-65 you reverse the aging process: bio-rejuvenation. TA-65 extends the telomeres and (thus) rejuvenates the cell, makes it 'younger'.

We are as old as our cells. But as I said, even when using TA-65 the use of these four supplements is highly recommended for the simple reason that you're filling up your bath with the drain wide open. Fine, but not optimal!

Chapter 39

Nocturnal leg cramps

Nocturnal legs cramps (not to be confused with restless legs, which are not painful) may occur at any age but are – like hearing loss- most - prevalent in the elderly (70+), as my own clinical experience bears out. As wiki correctly states the real cause is unknown and the cramps typically occur early in the morning (six o'clock) after hours of immobility. It gives a double whammy: you are rudely awakened from a deep sleep and the cramps are so excruciatingly painful that you must stumble out of bed on a 'wooden leg' and try, without falling over, to walk about until the cramp subsides. In some people being rudely awakened from a deep sleep - be it from a loud alarm or a painful cramp - spoils their day: their mind doesn't function normally, resulting in their 'quality of life' dropping from 8 to 4, in a manner of speech. Zwarte Riek (Black Rita, a well-known Dutch folk singer in Holland in the seventies) told me once that if she was rudely awakened by a loud alarm her whole day would be spoilt. Her mind couldn't function normally. Well something like that happens to me when I have had a night cramp.

What follows is a personal story with a very interesting universal outcome.

I started getting night cramps perhaps a decade ago. At first the usual measures like magnesium and quinine (Inhibin) worked fairly well. As I grew older they stopped being effective. Eventually nothing worked. I was at the mercy of these cramps which sometimes even occurred in the middle of the night. I was 'desperate', trying out even the silliest things, like going to a masseur and putting sunlight soap in my bed, a crazy measure suggested by several of my patients, including one of the hundred richest men in Holland, a smart entrepreneur (by the way, allow me a little boast: my son, Robert, is currently no 62 on the so called QUOTE 500 listing). In the fifties Ann Landers, the famous American health writer, was the first to suggest the use of sunlight soap in her daily column. Although my bed became a minefield of bars of soap my cramps continued unabated.

One day a patient of mine, a 72 year old elegant woman told me, "I've been using C60 (see chapter 42 for a month now and my night cramps are much better."

Vaguely, I had had the same impression since I started using C60 three months earlier. I increased the recommended daily dose ten-fold, mainly for longevity, and lo and behold two months later the cramps had virtually ceased. Which for me was a VERY BIG ISSUE for years is now no longer a problem. **The leg cramps are gone, which effectively means that a classical aging phenomenon has been eliminated**. In the light of the effect of C60 on aging and life–extension (chapter 41) this strongly suggests that C60 has eliminated this aging sign and thus – partly - rejuvenated the organism by several years, perhaps a decade.

If you suffer from nocturnal night cramps and magnesium or quinine is ineffective don't first try soap or the masseur but start using C60 right away. You will sleep longer and live longer …

Chapter 40

Irregular heartbeats and pig's heart valve: matters of the heart

This brief chapter, which deals with two heart problems that especially afflict **the older person**, is included because a) I personally suffer from irregular heartbeats (extra systoles) and b) because I'm taking a simple vitamin, K2, to prevent the calcification of a heart valve – a problem of the elderly – which often requires an operation.

Irregular heartbeats in the elderly
Let me start with a personal anecdote.
As a student I noted my heart skipping beats (extra systoles), a very unpleasant sensation. De cardiologist told me to stop smoking (8 a day) and lo and behold the rhythm normalized immediately. Some 30 years ago it started again (a very severe form which left me fatigued and feeling unwell for years). Q10, 100 mg, helped but the effective solution was a divorce! Purely psychological stress.
I'm currently 87 (2014) and have been suffering from 'skipping beats' (1 in 2) for about 6 months despite the use of Q10 for donkey's years. At the recommendation of a friend, a heart surgeon, I started using a beta-blocker, sotalol (80mg/day) which proved 'fairly effective' with unpredictable periods of irregular pulse throughout the day. Although these 'skipping beats' are not dangerous they are a nuisance, even if it were just because of the unpleasant drumbeats in your chest and sometimes feeling slightly unwell.
Currently I'm using 10-20 gram taurine powder (in two divided doses) in combination with 6 grams arginine powder on the basis of a 2006 scientific paper with the telling title '**Elimination of cardiac arrhythmias using oral taurine with L-arginine**' (Eby, G. and W.W. Halcomb, Medical Hypotheses, 67, 1200, 2006)

My pulse is very much better now and I'm feeling much better, including 'more energy'. By the way, the 'energizing effect' of Red Bull is not due to the caffeine but to the taurine content of the drink.

Just as a safety net I'm still using the beta-blocker, but thus far no more long periods of erratic heartbeats. One *caviat* is in order: 'too much' taurine may cause serious constipation in some people. Another warning: only rarely taurine helps in atrial fibrillation like in this patient reported in one of Dr. Eby's papers: 'The arrhythmias in the 60-year old male decreased dramatically (95-100 percent reduction) with elimination of heavy palpitations and atrial fibrillations upon addition of L-arginine to his taurine treatment. He remained symptom-free essentially all of the time.' (unquote).

> What is taurine? It is a naturally occurring (sulphur-containing) amino acid found in fish, meat, eggs. It is called a semi-essential amino acid, in contrast to the familiar essential amino acids used as building blocks for proteins.
>
> Our body is able to manufacture this amino acid but in the elderly this capacity declines. Vegetarians have a lower intake of taurine, whose daily intake via food ranges between 50-200 mg. So, the recommended daily dose for heart abnormalities is huge, but here it is used as a drug. Taurine is essential for normal heart functioning and the highest concentrations are found in the heart and in the retina.
>
> *Perhaps when you are suffering from atrial fibrillation it might be worth your while to try taurine (10-20 gram/day) in combination with L-arginine (6 grams/day). Beta-blockers (Sotalol) are often effective but a semi-permanent cure is ablation (see wiki) performed in a hospital with a lot of experience (at least 100 operations a year).*

Calcified aortic valve operation
As you grow older past 60 there always lurks the danger that your aortic valve will get calcified, leading to stenosis (narrowing) and insufficiency (regurgitation). Unless you want to go through life as a cripple an operation (usually open-heart surgery) will be required to replace the sick valve by a porcine valve or a mechanical one. If you're healthy, leading a healthy life style, this may happen only after 80, still a most unpleasant surprise with many risks at such an advanced age possibly leading to all sorts of post-operative complications including pneumonia which may kill you.

So, in order to avoid being stuck with a calcified aortic valve I'm taking vitamin K2 (the so-called MK-7 variant as a preventive measure.

Before proceeding it should be noted that in old age it is as if the calcium from the bones migrates to other parts of the body, leaving the bones 'decalcified' (osteoporosis) and the tissues calcified. As noted the gravest danger is, apart from calcified arteries, a calcified aortic valve.

Now vitamin K is a bit complicated (see Wiki). There are three forms, K1, K2 and K3.

Only K2 is of interest in this context. K2, or, menachinon (pronounced menakinon), abbreviated MK, exists in different flavours, MK-6, MK-7, etc.

For our purpose (don't get confused) only MK-7 is of interest as protection against aortic valve calcification.

By the way MK-7 is produced by bacteria during the fermentation of soya to produce natto, a favourite breakfast dish in Japan.

MK-7, heart valve and vessel wall calcification

MK-7 protects against calcification by activating the matrix-Gla-protein MGP (don't be alarmed), one of the strongest inhibitors of calcium deposition in the heart valve and vessel wall. When there is a shortage of K2 (MK-7) MGP is insufficiently active, resulting in progressive calcification, an insidious process.

As I aim to reach 100+ but dread to be confronted with open−heart surgery and a porcine valve I have been taking MK-7 (90 mcg) for years. I urge you to do the same. Always plan for the future, man; not only with regard to your pension!

A friend of mine, a doctor, had a valve replacement in his sixties. Perhaps he might have avoided it if he had taken MK-7 daily.

A more interesting case is discussed in Suzanne Somers', book Bombshell (2012), a collection of interviews with the leading giants in the life-extension field.

It concerns the famous life-extension guru, Jack LaLanne, who had written many books on health matters and aimed to reach 100+.

He died at 96 as a result of complications following a heart operation for a calcified aortic valve.

The following quote is taken from her interview with Dr. Bill Faloon, cofounder of the Life Extension Foundation, the largest longevity organisation in the world and publisher of Life Extension magazine which reports on cutting edge health and science issues (by the way, of course I'm a subscriber).

Bill Faloon: We aggressively sought out reasons why Jack LaLanne died at ninety-six considering his objectives of living well beyond one hundred years. From what we gather, his first major event occurred in 2009 when at the age of ninety-five he underwent aortic replacement surgery. A little over thirteen months later, he died at age ninety-six of respiratory failure due to pneumonia. Even in healthy elderly individuals, the impact of aortic valve surgery can be what we call the 'catastrophic pathological event' that leads to a downward spiral culminating in death. Jack was ahead of his time in so many ways, yet he appears to have missed out on one key nutrient-vitamin K2 that may have prevented *calcification* of his aortic valve.

Susanne Somers: So you are saying that he might be alive today had he taken vitamin K2 supplements?

Bill Faloon (abbrev.): It's hard to say, but a compelling volume of data substantiates the role of vitamin K2 in protecting against calcification throughout the body, so people who have not yet developed aortic stenosis can benefit enormously by taking it.

Suzanne Somers: So with everything Jack LaLanne did, the simple omission of vitamin K2, may have led to his dying whereas he could have lived even longer had he supplemented K2?

Bill Faloon: I'm afraid so. We fear that Jack LaLanne's *omission* of vitamin K2 may have created his catastrophic event that is, the aortic stenosis [narrowing] that predisposed him to pneumonia. (Unquote)

Let this case be a lesson if you aim at living well beyond 80. Be prepared and start taking MK-7 (a variant of K2) daily in a dose of 90 mcg or higher.

Life Extension Foundation (founded by Bill Faloon in 1980) (google) is a reliable source.

Chapter 41

The sleeping pill and eternal sleep

Let me start with a personal note. I've always been a 'poor' sleeper, but until some ten years ago I never took a sleeping pill (hypnotic). Since then I used to take a quart Temazepam 10 mg (so, 2.5 mg) at around 2 o'clock, (I wake up several times during the night) and regularly also an anti-histamine pill with sedative action, polaramine. I have stopped taking them some time ago. Why? Because I found a scientific paper from 2012 that sleeping pills (and sedative anti-histamines) greatly increase the risk of dying and increase the risk of cancer by 50 percent. That I'm still alive and well is a small miracle.

Although as many as 22 studies, including the Cancer Prevention Study of the American Cancer Society had earlier shown a link between increased mortality and the use of sleeping pills, professor D.F. Kripke's 2012 paper[66] in the leading medical journal *The British Medical Journal (BMJ)* provided the definitive proof of the high mortality linked to the use of sleeping pills. Dr. Kripke is the founder of the first *'sleep clinics'* in the United States (1973) and (co)author of hundreds of scientific papers about sleep disturbances and sleeping pills.

In this study over 10.000 people using sleeping pills were compared with a control group of over 20.000 matched individuals (with respect to age, life-style, etc.) during an observation period of 2.5 years.

It turned out that people who used more than 130 sleeping pills a year had more than six times the risk of dying. Perhaps even more disturbing is that people who only used a sleeping pill 18 times a

---

[66] D.F. Kripke et.al. *Hypnotics' association with mortality an cancer: a matched cohort study,* BMJ Open , 2012, Febr.27,2(1) e00850.

year had a greater than 3.5 times the 'normal' mortality risk. This relationship applied to all sleeping pills, including barbiturates, benzodiazepines (Temazepam, etc.) and newer drugs like Ambien, Sonata, etc. as well as sedative antihistamines (Polaramine).

Moreover, the cancer risk is increased by 35 percent if you use a sleeping pill more than 120 days a year.

Oh, what dreadful news! What's the alternative? Stop taking them?. But that would be awful . Then I would stay awake all night!

The reality is different for the vast majority of 'addicts'. Although the information leaflet, too, says you should use a sleeping pill only for a few weeks because of the risk of habituation and dependence, doctors often prescribe it for years at the patient's request. That makes sense, for otherwise the patient would simply seek another family doctor!

A large study sponsored by the National Institutes of Health (USA) that sleeping pills, including newer ones like Ambien, shorten the time before falling asleep by only 13 minutes and the total time of sleep by merely 11 minutes. When you compare this 'gain' with the greatly increased mortality and cancer risk you would be well advised to stop using them. Personally, I'm now 'clean' sleep -wise not wore off *and still alive*, thank goodness!

Suggestions

Here are some suggestions for better sleep:

- Try valerian, tryptophan or melatonin
- Take a hot bath or shower at bedtime
- If you're bothered by cold feet use socks or/and a hot water bottle
- Sleep in a really dark room or use a sleep mask and – if required - earplugs (Ohropax)
- No coffee after 4 o'clock
- No scary film or book before sleeping
- Consider a relaxation-CD (Google)
- If you wake up at night and stay widely awake get up and watch TV or read a book for a while

If you are a total insomniac do use a sleeping pill: chronic lack of sleep may shorten your life even more.

Chapter 42

C60 doubles the lifespan of rats

This may well be one of the shortest chapters, but one of the most important for your 'conservation': life-extension. It concerns a recent study on rats.(20012).[67]

In this study a doubling of (mean) life-span was achieved by regular oral administration of the substance C60 during 'middle age', i.e. from month 10 to month 17 (the mean life span of the rats is 24 months). This is unique, unheard of!

The aim of this experiment was not 'life-extension', but to test the chronic toxicity of C60.

The greatest life-extension that has thus far been achieved in test-animals (mammals) is about 30 percent, which is achieved by the drastic measure of (30 percent) calorie–restriction (see earlier chapters).

In human terms a life-extension of 90 percent (the official figure) means that the 'vitalist', who can live to be hundred today, may expect to reach the venerable age of 190 with C60. But you probably will have to start using C60 in middle-age.

Incidentally, although 6 rats were used in the experiment one rat who refused to die after living more than 120 percent longer than expected was prematurely killed because the researchers wanted to wrap up the experiment. If this one is included the average life-extension was 100 percent (rather than 90).

About 200 years for humans with C60 is only a 'theoretical' possibility, the more so because it is uncertain whether what holds for the rat will also apply to the human condition.

There is the rub. Roughly speaking it is estimated that what works in the rat works only in 90 percent of cases in man. To

---

[67] Baadi, T. et al: "The prolongation of lifespan of rats by repeated oral administration of [60] fullerene", Biomaterials, 33, 4936, 2012.

offer one negative example. A drug cutting off the blood supply to tumours works beautifully in rats (mice) but is ineffective in humans, prompting the Harvard professor, a surgeon, who developed the treatment, to declare, "If you're a rat I could cure you."

Bearing this *caviat* in mind you should still seriously consider using C60 because: a) it is harmless, b) in the rat experiment the quality of life is well maintained, c) the potential gain in life-expectancy is enormous and d) C60 is very cheap.

Of course I'm using C60 and hope to use it for many more years (I'm currently, 2014, 87)

For life-extension only C60 dissolved in olive oil and properly prepared is effective. A reliable address is www.c60antiaging.com

Pure C60 or C60 dissolved in water is unsuitable (toxic). Only C60 dissolved in oil (olive-oil) which then has to undergo a special procedure is effective.

Currently (2014) a good review (Google) is: **Buckyballs, health and longevity-state of affairs.** It is the website of the academic Vince Guliano, a 'genius'.

Point by point I present a number of relevant aspects of C60.

- The rats in the placebo group died of cancer (80 percent) or of pneumonia (weak immune system).
  The rats in the treated group (C60) did not get cancer and died – after living twice longer – not from a disease but from 'old age': massive organ failure (liver, heart, kidneys), because the telomeres had reached their critical length (Chapter 13).
  Important lesson: C60 (probably also in humans) is the most important defence against cancer. This conclusion is supported by a wealth of direct evidence. For example the growth and dissemination of human cancers implanted in mice are greatly inhibited by C60 administration. C60 also inhibits the growth of (human) cancer cells in *vitro* (grown in the lab).

- C6o stimulates hair growth in test animals by revitalizing the hair follicles. C60 also promotes the hair growth in human skin grown in the laboratory.
  In humans, too, it promotes hair growth and hair quality (fuller, shinier).
  Personal note: my hairdresser noted after I had been using C60 for only a month, that my hair was fuller and better (blind observer).

- C60 is a molecule consisting of 60 carbon atoms in the shape of a ball which is structurally identical to the classic football (five-angle and six -angle). It is like a cage that can contain atoms or small molecules.
  By the way pure carbon can exist in 3 forms: 1) diamond (crystal), 2) graphene (flat 'two-dimensional' sheets like chicken wire; pencil (graphite) consists of these sheets stacked together, and 3) C60, football-shaped, better known as Bucky balls, after the famous architect Buckminster Fuller, the scientists who discovered C60 and synthesized it. He received the Nobel prize in 1985.

- C60 nearly is completely excreted via the bile in 24 hours.

- Translating the rat experiment to the human condition the following theoretical picture emerges. Suppose 100 male subjects start using C60 from the age of 40 to the age of 50 (so, after that, no more) The average lifespan of males in the Netherlands is 80 years. The men who used C60 only for ten years then go on living until they reach 160 years on the average. In excellent shape and without cancer!
  How would that be possible? The scientists are perplexed. But the facts have the last word (at least for the rat: living 100 percent longer and without cancer, the scourge of mankind to which at least one in three succumb during their lifetime and which is a major cause of death in old age. Another scourge of old age is Alzheimer's disease. Here too C60 may be protective

as the medically–grounded reader may deduce from the title of a 2012 paper entitled, *"Fullerene [C60] prevents neurotoxicity induced by intrahippocampal microinjection of amyloid beta peptides"*.

For a full discussion the reader is referred to Guiliano's website mentioned above.

Let me end this paragraph on a personal note
Since in the rat experiment C60 was dissolved in olive oil there was - apart from the 'control group' - another set of rats who received only the solvent (olive oil), without the C60.

Surprise, surprise: the rats receiving only the olive oil lived on the average 18 percent longer than the rats in the control group.

Amazing. Not on scientific grounds, but as a kind of Dr. Watson (Sherlock Holmes) and 'vitalist' I now use olive oil daily (50 ml), partly in the salad and partly 'pure'. Why? Solely because of the 18 percent? No, also because there are many intriguing indications that it may be life-extender in man too. It is of some interest to note that the oldest person ever, Jeanne Calment (122), consumed large amounts of olive oil daily, even for French standards, while for example farmers in Crete, who daily consume over 100 ml olive oil live, on the average. remarkably long lives, as you may verify by visiting the local cemeteries.

Medical note
Nobody knows how C60 exerts its life-extending action. Currently the most plausible theory (hypothesis) is that C60 favourably affects DNA methylation and DNA repair (Guiliano-Watson hypothesis). It is known that C60 acts as a powerful and inexhaustible ('recycling') mitochondrial antioxidant and strengthens the microtubule networks in the cell, the transport system of the cell.

Also, since C60 (at least in rats) extends life beyond the maximal life span of the species, and as both theoretical calculations and direct evidence support the view that maximal lifespan is determined by telomere shrinkage to 'critical length', it follows that C60 must also slow down telomere shortening, possibly through its powerful antioxidant action (von Zglinicki).

Chapter 43

Bad marriage, bad health

Indeed, science also probes into your private life. It has found that a good marriage is good for your health and vice versa. As early as the sixties professor J.J. Groen had shown that men in a bad marriage (cold, heartless wife) had a greatly increased risk of getting a heart attack. A recent Swedish study showed that women in a bad marriage with an existing heart condition had a three times greater risk of serious cardiac complications.

Marriage problems increase the production of stress hormones like adrenaline and cortisol (chapter 30), resulting in elevated blood pressure, cardiac overload, weakened immune system, etc.

As I mentioned earlier in my book *Stress without Stress,* the well-known British scientist and clinical psychologist professor Hans Eysenck showed in a 10-year study that chronic stress (including marriage stress) resulted in a 40 percent increase in mortality. The stressed individual may die, depending on his personality structure (type A, etc.) from either an infarction (heart, stroke) or cancer. Both men and women in a bad marriage with much animosity and fighting were shown to have considerably more calcification in the major arteries and heart than the control group, as shown by CT scan.

As early as the sixties a study showed that students who were in love had far fewer colds than their peers. Love strengthens the immune system. Hate (bad marriage) does the reverse.

The number of studies on relation stress and health (illness) runs into the hundreds. But I'll not bother you any further with scientific findings.

One thing is certain. **No company is better than bad company.**

But do you have to file for a divorce when your marriage is not up to par? Of course not. Try to find a 'peaceful' solution. Recently a couple whom I had known for many years told me in my office that they had been on the point of separating. Suddenly the weather had changed: flaming quarrels, geysers of hate. At the last moment they decided to seek the help of a marriage counsellor. Calm has been restored, divorce is off.

But if tensions remain high, enmity rules, warmth is totally lacking, you have to ask yourself for the sake of your own health and well-being, 'Can this marriage still be saved or should I put an end to it?' Children and finances may pose an enormous obstacle. Each case is unique and cutting the Gordian knot is in most cases, as has been shown by an American study, just a matter of the last straw: the last of many quarrels. Indeed 'the straw that broke the camel's back'.